Guru Yoga

According to the Preliminary Practice of Longchen Nyingtik

Guru Yoga

According to the Preliminary Practice of Longchen Nyingtik

An Oral Teaching by
Dilgo Khyentse Rinpoche

Translated by
Matthieu Ricard
(Gelong Könchog Tenzin)

Edited by
Rigpa

Snow Lion Publications
Ithaca, New York

Snow Lion Publications
P.O. Box 6483
Ithaca, New York 14851 U.S.A.
Telephone: 607-273-8519

www.snowlionpub.com

Printed in Canada on acid-free recycled paper.

ISBN 1-55939-121-9

Library of Congress Cataloging-in-Publication Data

Rab-gsal-zla-ba, Dis-mgo Mkhyen-brtse, 1910-
Guru Yoga : according to the preliminary practice of Longchen Nyingtik : an oral teaching by Dilgo Khyentse Rinpoche / translated by Matthieu Ricard (Gelong Könchog Tenzin) ; edited by Rigpa.
p. cm.
ISBN 1-55939-121-9
1. Guru worship (Rite)—Buddhism. 2. Rdzogs-chen (Rñiṅ-ma-pa) I. Rigpa. II. Title.

BQ7662.6.R34 1999
294.3'4446—dc21

Contents

Dedication

For the reincarnation of Dilgo Khyentse Rinpoche, Urgyen Tenzin Jigme Lhundrup, for all the teachers who are Khyentse Rinpoche's disciples, and for all the masters of the Longchen Nyingtik lineage: may their lives be long and their enlightened activity fill the world!

May Khyentse Rinpoche's wisdom, compassion, and power come to touch and transform the lives of people everywhere, and may his glorious vision and aspirations be fulfilled!

Foreword

Why do we practice Guru Yoga, "union with the nature of the guru"? With the help of the outer teacher, we can discover the inner teacher—the nature of our own mind. Until we reach that point, if we seriously wish to transform ourselves, we should never be overconfident and rely solely on our own methods and our own experience. The path can only be trodden by ourselves, using our own effort, yet even so we can never dispense with the advice of an experienced guide. To give that guidance is the role of the spiritual teacher.

We have had the immense good fortune to meet extraordinary masters like Khyentse Rinpoche, who, without any doubt, possessed all the qualities of an authentic spiritual teacher. Such teachers are increasingly rare. It is of crucial importance to choose a teacher wisely, making sure that his qualities are attuned to those of the perfect masters of the past.

In my own case, I saw Khyentse Rinpoche at first as a most loving and wonderful grandfather. Then, gradually, my affection for him turned into a deep, unchanging devotion as I came to see him as my root master and spiritual guide. He is constantly in my thoughts, inspiring every instant of my life through his enlightened and compassionate presence.

Guru Yoga should be at the heart of every practice we do. It gives our practice strength and depth, and prevents us from straying into all the side-tracks dreamed up by our wild thoughts. The very essence of Buddhist practice is to destroy ego-clinging, totally—and the most inspiring way to do that is through the practice of Guru Yoga.

Shechen Rabjam Rinpoche

Introduction

Any spiritual history of the 20th century would be incomplete without paying tribute to Kyabjé Dilgo Khyentse Rinpoche (1910–1991), a figure of undisputed greatness, whose influence and inspiration have touched countless thousands of people around the world. He belonged to the last generation of spiritual masters trained in Tibet, whose lives bore that same stamp of depth and mystery and singularity of purpose as those of the great Asian, European, and Middle Eastern saints and mystics of the past. The teacher of so many of the Tibetan masters of today, including His Holiness the Dalai Lama, Khyentse Rinpoche came, in the eyes of the Buddhist world, to personify the very archetype of a guru, his name a byword for authenticity and integrity, and for everything that was good and noble about Tibet and its Buddhist heritage. By simply being who he was, he naturally defined the criteria for what a great lama should be.

Much has been written in recent times about Khyentse Rinpoche and his extraordinary life, a life dedicated entirely to the welfare of others and to nourishing the life-force of the ancient teachings of Buddha. And there is so much to tell: his recognition, when young, as the mind emanation of Jamyang

Khyentse Wangpo; his twenty-two years in retreat; his studies with over fifty legendary teachers; his devotion to his masters, particularly Shechen Gyaltsap and Jamyang Khyentse Chökyi Lodrö; his amazing learning and deep realization; his revelation of the treasures of Padmasambhava; his twenty-five volumes of poetic and inspired writings; his great achievements in building, restoration, and publishing; his seemingly superhuman energy and tireless compassion; the captivating beauty and completeness of his spoken teachings; the unique and effortless manner in which he taught and passed on the transmissions and teachings he held in such great number; and his travels all over the Himalayas, India, Tibet, Southeast Asia, and the West to teach his thousands of disciples. That one human being could have achieved so much in one lifetime is almost inconceivable.

Khyentse Rinpoche was a teacher of the highest spiritual attainment, and yet, as all who knew or met him will say, a person of the most tender and disarming warmth and kindness. Head of the Nyingma School and a supreme master of Dzogpachenpo, he was a champion of the "Rimé" nonsectarian spirit, which was revealed in his remarkable ability to transmit the teachings of each lineage according to its own tradition. He carried forward the enlightened vision and ideals of the 19th-century pioneers of the Rimey movement, Jamyang Khyentse Wangpo (1820–1892), Jamgön Kongtrul (1813–1899), and Chokgyur Lingpa (1829–1870), playing a vital role in the reconstruction of Tibetan Buddhist spiritual life and culture after the shattering blows of the Tibetan holocaust. Sometimes it is difficult to imagine that a master of his calibre will ever be seen again, and yet one thing is certain: if there *are* other masters who follow in his footsteps, or who even begin to emulate his greatness, then it will be thanks to him and to the care and attention he gave to the future survival of the Buddhist teachings, and especially the Nyingma lineage, as a living tradition of realization. And he ensured its continuity in all kinds of ways. In December 1997, his reincarnation, Urgyen Tenzin Jigme Lhundrup, born in 1993 on the anniversary of Guru Padmasambhava's birth, was enthroned at Shechen Monastery in Nepal.

The teachings on Guru Yoga presented in this book were themselves given during an extraordinary and historic occasion. No one who was there could ever forget those days during the summer of 1984 in Dordogne in France, when both Kyabjé Dudjom Rinpoche and Kyabjé Dilgo Khyentse Rinpoche—the two most eminent masters of the Nyingma tradition, the living representatives of Padmasambhava, and peerless exponents of Dzogpachenpo—taught to about five hundred practitioners who had come from all over the world. In the mornings Dudjom Rinpoche gave what was to be his last public teaching, on the practice of Dzogchen from Padmasambhava's famous *Prayer in Seven Chapters;* in the afternoons Dilgo Khyentse Rinpoche granted empowerments and gave teachings at his residence, La Sonnerie. Many other masters of the Nyingma tradition who were their students gathered there, including Nyoshul Khen Rinpoche, Shechen Rabjam Rinpoche, Pema Wangyal Rinpoche, Jigme Khyentse Rinpoche, Shenphen Rinpoche, and Sogyal Rinpoche, as well as five great ḍākinis, the spiritual consorts of Jamyang Khyentse Chökyi Lodrö, Dudjom Rinpoche, Dilgo Khyentse Rinpoche, Kangyur Rinpoche, and Nyoshul Khen Rinpoche.

It was during those long August afternoons, the gathering assembled on the lawn at La Sonnerie, with the sunlight slanting down through the trees, that Khyentse Rinpoche gave these teachings on Guru Yoga at the request of Sogyal Rinpoche and Rigpa, who were holding their annual summer retreat nearby. This particular Guru Yoga, called *The Wish-fulfilling Jewel,* is the outer practice of the guru from the Longchen Nyingtik revelation of the visionary master Rigdzin Jikmé Lingpa (1730–1798). It forms the climax to the Ngöndro preliminary practice of Longchen Nyingtik, entitled the *Excellent Path to Omniscience,* which was compiled by Jikmé Lingpa's great disciple, Dodrupchen Jikmé Trinlé Özer.

Jikmé Lingpa's immediate incarnation was Jamyang Khyentse Wangpo, whose own incarnation was Dilgo

Khyentse Rinpoche, a lineage holder of the Longchen Nyingtik. Who better, then, to give this teaching, and especially one who, for so many, had come to exemplify and embody the guru? As the Dalai Lama wrote:

> Khyentse Rinpoche was a model for all other holders of the teachings. We should not only admire his inconceivable knowledge, wisdom and accomplishment, but, more importantly, we should follow his example and emulate those qualities ourselves... Deep spiritual experiences, which seem to transcend logical explanation, are not easily expressed in words or transmitted by means of verbal explanation. They depend, rather, on the inspiration and blessings received from the spiritual lineage through one's teacher. This is why in Buddhism (and particularly Vajrayāna Buddhism), the practice of Guru Yoga—"union with the teacher's nature"—is given such great importance. This is all the more so for the realization of awareness, *rigpa*, in the Great Perfection (Dzogchen) tradition. Since the practice of Guru Yoga is so important, the qualities of the teacher himself are extremely important too. The qualities necessary for an authentic teacher were described in great detail by the Buddha himself in many sūtras and tantras. All of these qualities I found in Khyentse Rinpoche.[1]

A teacher who quite naturally inspired devotion, Khyentse Rinpoche would constantly emphasize the importance of Guru Yoga, particularly with regard to the transmission and practice of Dzogchen. According to the approach of Dzogchen, the wisdom mind of the master can actually be realized, not simply through study and practice, but through an uncontrived and heartfelt devotion; Khyentse Rinpoche used to illustrate this through the story of the origin of the Longchen Nyingtik.

The cycle of Longchen Nyingtik, "The Heart Essence of Infinite Expanse," a collection of tantras and sādhanas, was discovered by Jikmé Lingpa as a mind treasure.[2] An overwhelming awe and devotion had been awakened in him by reading the teachings of Longchen Rabjam (1308–1363), the exceptional master and genius who had synthesized and clarified the Dzogchen teachings in a series of brilliant writings. At the age of thirty-one, Jikmé Lingpa undertook a three-year retreat in the Chimphu caves, near Samyé. He prayed to Longchen Rabjam with such fervor that, although they were separated by some four hundred years, Longchen Rabjam appeared to him in his wisdom body on three occasions, granting him the blessing of his body, speech, and wisdom mind. This encounter was of extraordinary moment. It released in Jikmé Lingpa boundless wisdom and the highest realization of Dzogpa-chenpo, and empowered him to transmit and teach the Longchen Nyingtik.

In his *Treasury of Precious Qualities,* Jikmé Lingpa wrote, "the supreme disciple is the one with supreme devotion," and he became renowned, in fact, as a master who attained tremendous learning without much study, but through profound meditation and through intense devotion. This, Khyentse Rinpoche used to say, was the auspicious precedent and tradition of the Longchen Nyingtik lineage, a lineage forever marked by unwavering devotion. Because they inherited this special lineage, Jamyang Khyentse Wangpo and Patrul Rinpoche both treasured this particular Guru Yoga as the heart of their practice. Devotion is what led to the revelation of the Longchen Nyingtik, it is what has characterized the lineage ever since, and it is what has guided its remarkable spread, to become one of the most popular and widespread cycles of Dzogchen teachings, both in Tibet and the Himalayas, and now in the western world.

The Guru Yoga teachings here were translated orally by Ven. Könchog Tenzin, Matthieu Ricard, who spent more than twelve years as Khyentse Rinpoche's assistant. Matthieu then edited the entire text in 1990, during Khyentse Rinpoche's final visit to France, when he gave teachings and empowerments to one thousand five hundred people at the request of Sogyal Rinpoche and Rigpa, at Prapoutel, near Grenoble.

Perhaps there is no one better suited to introduce this book on Guru Yoga than Shechen Rabjam Rinpoche, Dzongsar Khyentse Rinpoche, Dzigar Kongtrul Rinpoche, and Tsikey

Chokling Rinpoche. Shechen Rabjam Rinpoche, who wrote the foreword, is Khyentse Rinpoche's grandson and Dharma-heir. Dzongsar Khyentse Rinpoche, Dzigar Kongtrul Rinpoche, and Tsikey Chokling Rinpoche, who contributed the preface, are three of Khyentse Rinpoche's closest disciples; they are the present-day incarnations of Jamyang Khyentse Wangpo, Jamgön Kongtrul, and Chokgyur Lingpa, whose collaboration played such a huge part in shaping the Tibetan Buddhism we know today.

Preface

How fortunate we are to be able to read a teaching like this on Guru Yoga by Dilgo Khyentse Rinpoche, who is actually the great master Longchen Rabjam in person. The Longchen Nyingtik has been treasured by all the great Khyentses of the past as their most important inner practice. Nowadays, when genuine devotion for the guru is rare because most of us lack the necessary wisdom and merit, to be able to receive this teaching from such a master is an extraordinary blessing.

The purpose of Dharma practice is to attain enlightenment. Actually, attaining enlightenment is exactly the same as ridding ourselves of ignorance, and the root of ignorance is the ego. Whichever path we take, whether it's the long and disciplined route, or the short and wild one, at the end of it the essential point is that we eliminate the ego.

There are many, many different ways we can do this, for example through Śamatha meditation, and they all work to one extent or another. However, since we have been with our ego for so many lifetimes and we are so familiar with it, every time we take to a path in our efforts to eliminate ego, that very path is hijacked by ego and manipulated in such a way that rather than crushing the ego, our path only helps to reinforce it.

This is the reason why, in the Vajrayāna, guru devotion, or Guru Yoga, is taught as a vital and essential practice. As the guru is a living, breathing human being, he or she is able to deal directly with your ego. Reading a book about how to eliminate ego may be interesting, but you will never be in awe of that book, and anyway, books are entirely open to your own interpretation. A book cannot talk or react to you, whereas the guru can and will stir up your ego so that eventually it will be eliminated altogether. Whether this is achieved wrathfully or gently doesn't matter, but in the end this is what the guru is there to do, and this is why guru devotion is so important.

For a student who has true devotion, the guru is the embodiment of all sources of refuge, and devotion for the guru is the essence of all paths. Lama Jamyang Gyaltsen, a great Sakyapa master, said, "The guru is the embodiment of all refuge," meaning that when we take refuge, we see the guru present in all of the Three Jewels: the guru's physical presence is seen as the Saṅgha, the guru's teaching is seen as the Dharma, and the guru's mind is seen as the Buddha.

Guru Yoga is the quickest, most effective method for attaining enlightenment and is the one path in which all other paths are complete. Guru Yoga includes renunciation, bodhicitta, development (Kyérim) and completion (Dzogrim) meditation, and mind training (Lojong), which is why we can say that Guru Yoga is the embodiment, or the essence, of all paths. It is the key to them all, the special method that can take a practitioner through the stages of the bodhisattva path and the different Yānas. Other paths can take you to a certain level, but they are not complete. Guru Yoga is not only the complete path, but also the most condensed.

In order to practice Guru Yoga, first we must learn how to see our guru as the Buddha. In our day-to-day lives, even if we have a guru, we tend to look elsewhere for the solution to our problems. On an outer level, when we are ill we "take refuge" in a doctor, or if it's raining we "take refuge" in an umbrella. Similarly, on an inner level, if we have money problems we may try to solve them with Jambhala practice, if we face obstacles and difficulties we may invoke the help of

Mahākāla, or if we lack wisdom we may pray to Mañjuśrī. This shows how weak our devotion is, because whatever it is we lack, we need only look to one source for help and guidance: the guru. The first stage of guru devotion, then, is to awaken and enhance our devotion, until it becomes sound and strong and we can actually look upon the guru as the Buddha.

Gradually we will reach the second stage, where we don't simply *think* the guru is the Buddha, we *see* he is the Buddha. As our devotion becomes stronger still, it is with a growing sense of joy that we begin to rely entirely on the guru for everything. An inner confidence arises, an absolute certainty that the guru is the only source of refuge. No longer do we have to create or fabricate our devotion—now it comes quite naturally.

Then, all our experiences, good or bad, are manifestations of the guru. Everything we experience in life becomes beneficial and has a purpose; everything we encounter becomes a teaching. Total trust and devotion for the guru is born within our heart, and the blessing of the guru dissolves into our mind.

With this, we reach the third stage, which is when we realize that our mind is none other than the guru whom we have seen as the Buddha. Finally we have managed to merge our mind with the guru's mind, which takes us beyond all our ordinary habits of exaggeration and underestimation, and frees us from all sorts of expectation and fear. Our devotion is, at last, neither created nor fabricated but a true devotion, and once having achieved it, we will have realized the ultimate goal of all Buddhist practice.

Dzongsar Jamyang Khyentse Rinpoche

I do Guru Yoga every day. For me personally, Guru Yoga practice inspires me the most, and brings me in touch with my deepest nature. It also satisfies me the most; it makes me have no uncertainty about what I am doing with my life. That is really true—that much I can say.

Dzigar Kongtrul Rinpoche

Dilgo Khyentse Rinpoche was a siddha. He followed a great number of masters and attained the highest degree of learning in most fields of knowledge. For us, he was an embodiment of the original wakefulness of all buddhas, the lord of all maṇḍalas—a master who was indivisible from the mind of Padmasambhava. His heart was at peace in his compassionate resolve to liberate all beings. And it was this resolve that showed itself in the immense turning of the Wheel of Dharma he manifested throughout his life.

Concerning Guru Yoga, there are outer, inner, and innermost types of masters. The outer master is the one who explains to us the general points of spiritual practice, and how to begin the fourfold 100,000 preliminary practices. The inner master is the one who gives us Vajrayāna empowerment and explains the meaning of the tantras, and how to implement the tantric teachings in our lives. The innermost master is the one who gives us the pointing-out instruction, who brings us face to face with the naked state of non-dual awareness, so that we realize it in actuality within our own experience. In this way, the guru awakens the buddha from within our heart.

It is taught that, compared to making offerings to all the buddhas of the ten directions, there is more merit in making offerings to a single hair in one pore of the guru's body. So persevere in Guru Yoga. It is through the sincere practice of Guru Yoga that your three poisons subside, that boundless samādhi unfolds, and inconceivable benefits result; so definitely practice Guru Yoga!

Chokling Rinpoche, The 4th Tsikey Chokling,
Mingyur Dewey Dorje Trinley Kunkyab

The Turning Point

There is not a single sentient being who, over the course of our past lives, has not been our mother or father and so treated us with enormous kindness. Instead of discriminating, then, between enemies and loved ones, it should be quite natural for us to have the same feeling of love for all beings as we have for our parents in this life. Each and every one of them, without exception, wishes only to find happiness, and yet, blinded by ignorance, they fail to recognize that the true cause of that happiness is to accomplish the Dharma. Equally, there is not one of them who wants to suffer, and yet they do not recognize that the very cause of their suffering is negative actions. Simply reflecting on this will cause a great wave of compassion to surge up inside our minds.

However, a mere feeling of compassion on its own is not sufficient to help all beings actually reach the supreme level of enlightenment. Right now we have obtained this precious human body, we have met a qualified teacher, and by receiving his instructions we have crossed the threshold of the Dharma. So we find ourselves at a turning point—we can either go up or go down. Our principal motivation now must be the wish to establish all beings in complete enlightenment.

Yet, at the same time, we need to acknowledge that at present we simply do not possess the ability to free beings from saṃsāra. Therefore it is essential for us first of all to perfect our inner potential, along with all its qualities. It is with this kind of supreme attitude—one aimed at the benefit of all sentient beings—that we should endeavor with all our strength to receive the teachings, reflect on them, and put them into practice.

What practice can we do, then, to liberate all beings, to bring them to the highest level of enlightenment? At the moment, we have this most precious human body, which is not just some ordinary physical body, but the perfect support. It is endowed with eight freedoms from unfavorable conditions, and ten advantages or favorable conditions,[3] and so it is known as the "jewel-like human body." It is this which gives us the freedom to practice the Dharma.

However, to have this body is, by itself, not enough. We need to use it straightaway to practice the Dharma, for death may strike at any moment. One fact we must realize is how all phenomena—both the outer universe and all the beings within it—are utterly impermanent. They pass like a flash of lightning striking through the sky, or like a waterfall rushing down, without an instant's pause. Just as the outer universe changes with the passing of the seasons, so from morning to evening, from moment to moment, the same holds true for human beings. It says in the sūtras:

> Whatever is born will die,
> Whatever is gathered will be dispersed,
> Whatever is joined together will come apart,
> Whatever is high will be brought low.

This is why we should seize the opportunity of this human life now, so as to practice towards enlightenment, instead of squandering it, entangled in worldly affairs and preoccupations, always seeking to outdo our enemies and protect our kin, or look after our business affairs, land, and property. There we are, engrossed in all these activities, when suddenly death strikes us down. It will be too late then to practice the Dharma.

However beautiful you are, you will never beguile the Lord of Death. However rich you may be, you can never buy even one moment of life. However much power and influence you command, all your wealth and all your worldly achievements will in the end be utterly useless. Only the Dharma can help at the time of death.

Although it is a crucial point, simply to remember death is not enough; now that we have good health and freedom in both body and mind, we need to channel all our energy into practicing the Dharma. We should check, day after day, that we are not wasting our lives and that we are making every effort to blend the Dharma—the priceless instructions of the teacher—with our mindstream.

If we are able to do this and we are the best kind of practitioner, then at the time of death we shall be free from all fear and recognize the dharmakāya, the absolute nature. If we are a middling practitioner, we shall have the confidence of knowing that we will not be deluded by any of the phenomena that appear in the *bardo* state, and that we will then be able to achieve enlightenment. And if we are the most ordinary kind of practitioner, at the very least we will be free from regret, because we will be confident we have done our best to practice the Dharma, and therefore we will not take rebirth in the lower realms, but find the support we need in the next life to continue our Dharma practice.

What we must realize is that at the moment of death we are plucked from this life like a hair drawn from a piece of butter, leaving everything behind, including this body we have held so dear. Death is not like a fire that simply goes out, or like water that vanishes when it lands on dry ground. There will be rebirth, and this rebirth will be conditioned by our positive and negative actions. If we have accumulated negative actions, we will be reborn in the lower realms. However much we long to be reborn in the celestial realms, unless we have prepared for this by accumulating positive actions, it will be quite impossible. As it is said: "There is no result that we have experienced that was not created by past actions, and there is not a single present action that will not bear fruit." So we should never feel contempt towards accumulating even the smallest amount of merit and virtue, because the results can be enormous. Nor should we ever think that if we indulge in only a tiny negative action it is of little or no significance.

Following an authentic teacher and having received his instructions, we have to discriminate with great care between what is to be avoided and what is to be adopted, realizing that negative actions are the very cause of our ceaseless wandering in saṃsāra.

This is why we need to ensure that all our actions are governed by the Three Noble Principles. First is the preparation, which is the generation of bodhicitta—the wish to carry out whatever actions or accomplish whatever practice we can for the sake of all sentient beings. This links our practice with the supreme skillful means. Second is the actual practice, which is one-pointed concentration, free from any clinging. This renders our practice invulnerable to obstacles. Third is the conclusion, the dedication of all our merit for the good of all beings. This causes the merit of our practice to continue increasing until enlightenment. The very highest way of dedicating meritorious and positive actions is to do so for the enlightenment of all beings.

With these Three Noble Principles as our guide, we should constantly endeavor to cultivate goodness. We may amass all kinds of worldly virtue and merit, which may bring us temporary results like long life or wealth, but one day the fruit of all this merit will be exhausted, and we will plunge yet again into the lower realms. Even though the followers of the Fundamental Vehicle, the Śrāvakas and Pratyekabuddhas,[4] can free themselves from saṃsāra, it takes an extremely long time, many aeons in fact, for them to reach buddhahood. Through the supreme path of the Mahāyāna, the bodhisattvas' Great Vehicle, we can attain buddhahood swiftly, for the sake and benefit of all others.

If we truly wish to find freedom from this ocean of suffering, nothing could be more vital than to seek a correct, universal, and ultimate source of refuge. But first, we need to recognize the *nature* of saṃsāra because until and unless we realize that saṃsāra is totally pervaded by suffering, a strong sense of renunciation will never arise in our minds. We will only go on thinking that saṃsāra is enjoyable, and the thought of wanting to escape from it will never even occur to us. This is why it is so important to reflect deeply on saṃsāra and to realize that we are caught up in it like people trapped in the confines of a prison. There is no way that a prisoner can possibly escape by means of his or her own strength, but only by appealing for help from someone in a position of greater power. In exactly the same way, we need the aid of someone who has gone beyond saṃsāra.

We might wonder, "When did saṃsāra begin?" No one except an omniscient buddha could point and say, "This is the beginning of saṃsāra." The delusion perpetuated in saṃsāra's ocean of suffering has gone on throughout an infinite series of lives, and will continue for aeons if we do not do something to remedy it. As the Buddha said in the *Sūtra of Close Mindfulness*:

> If we were to pile up the limbs of all the insects
> Which had been our bodies in past lives,
> They would make a mountain higher than Mount Meru.

What ordinary beings fail to recognize is that saṃsāra is nothing but suffering. They are like people afflicted with an eye condition that causes them to see a white conch shell as yellow. However hard they look, they will never see it as white.

Three main types of suffering prevail in saṃsāra: suffering upon suffering, suffering of change, and all-pervasive suffering. "Suffering upon suffering" is when one experience of suffering comes right on top of another. A good example would be the continuously renewed suffering endured in the hells and other lower realms. "The suffering of change" is the constant change and fluctuation that takes place between fleeting states of happiness and suffering. Enjoyment, wealth, or fame may come our way, but they never last. Say, for instance, one lovely summer's day we go on a picnic with our friends. One moment we are sitting there on the grass, relaxed, carefree and contented, and then suddenly we are bitten by a snake. This is the suffering of change. "All-pervasive suffering" indicates that suffering pervades saṃsāra in its entirety and is always latent within it. Even those who dwell absorbed in states of deep samādhi on the higher planes of existence, like the formless celestial beings, do not escape suffering. When their karma and the fruits of their concentration are exhausted, they will fall once again into the lower realms, because their inner poisons have not been eradicated.

What refuge can we seek for protection and freedom from this ocean of suffering? Ordinary objects of refuge such as mountains, stars, natural forces, or powerful individuals, which are not free from saṃsāra themselves, cannot offer us enduring and universal protection. They can only disappoint us. The one and only supreme and infallible source of refuge—the one which is utterly free from any partiality, free from all attachment or rejection, and which possesses a universal compassion towards all beings—is the Three Jewels: the Buddha, the Dharma, and the Saṅgha.

The Buddha manifests as the three kāyas and five wisdoms, which comprise all the qualities of having discarded whatever is to be discarded, and having realized whatever is to be realized. The Dharma is the teaching given by the Buddha, which shows the path and leads to the cessation of suffering. The Saṅgha is the virtuous community, endowed with all the noble qualities of understanding and liberation.

On the innermost level, the Three Jewels are all gathered within the lama, or guru: his body is the Saṅgha, his speech is the Dharma, and his mind is the Buddha. He is like a wish-fulfilling jewel, the unerring union of all sources of refuge, his absolute nature beyond the intellectual mind. To remember the guru is the same as thinking of all the buddhas. This is why, if we rely on him totally, just this in itself will embrace the entire meaning and purpose of refuge.

Then, the principal path towards enlightenment is the generation of bodhicitta. Up until now we have segregated enemies and friends, those whom we wish to reject and those whom we wish to attract. But now we should think of all beings, without any discrimination, as being like our very own parents who have shown us the very greatest kindness. And if we stop to think about how kind our parents have been to us—how they clothed us, fed us, and devoted all of their time to our benefit and well-being—then our natural response and desire will be only to show our gratitude.

All beings wish to achieve happiness and avoid suffering, but because they do not know how to do so, all they succeed in doing is causing themselves more suffering. Everything they do runs counter to the fulfillment of their wishes. In order to free them all from suffering and lead them to enlightenment, we must not only arouse a strong feeling of compassion for them in our minds, but also we must act upon it and strive to put it into practice through the six perfections. The six perfections are: giving with generosity, maintaining discipline, meditating on patience, endeavoring with diligence, resting in equanimity, and realizing egolessness through the wisdom of discernment.

Guru Yoga

Of all practices, the one which, through its blessings, will fulfil our aims and aspirations most rapidly is Guru Yoga (or *Lamé Naljor* in Tibetan). Guru Yoga literally means "union with the nature of the guru" and it is both the quintessence and the ground of all the preliminary and main practices. It is the ultimate teaching, yet one which can be accomplished equally by anyone, whatever their capacity—superior, medium, or ordinary. For dispelling obstacles, making progress in our practice, and receiving blessings, there is no better practice than Guru Yoga. And it is as a result of the blessings obtained through practicing Guru Yoga that we can progress through the main practice—the development and completion stages, or Kyérim and Dzogrim—and so on to Dzogpachenpo.

Guru Yoga is the essence of the eighty-four thousand sections of Lord Buddha's teachings. It is said that all the buddhas of the past, present, and future have attained, and will attain, buddhahood through following an authentic spiritual teacher. To rely upon a qualified guru is the true way of a bodhisattva. According to the Secret Mantrayāna, Guru Yoga is the heart essence of the practice, and is treasured as the core of all practices in all lineages. In the Kagyü lineage, for example, one of the main practices is called "Carrying Devotion to the Guru along the Path," and in their pith instructions the greatest emphasis is laid on fervent devotion. The same holds true for the Sakya and Nyingma lineages as well.

There are many methods for accomplishing the three kāyas of the guru, and there are practices which focus on the guru on outer, inner, secret, and most secret levels.[5] Suffice it to say that Guru Yoga is the easiest to practice and yet the most profound. Here we are approaching it within the context of the Ngöndro preliminary practice of Longchen Nyingtik, known as *Nam Khyen Lam Zang*, or "The Excellent Path to Omniscience." The preliminary practice has six parts: the four thoughts which turn the mind from saṃsāra; taking refuge; the generation of bodhicitta; the purification through Vajrasattva; offering of the maṇḍala; and finally, Guru Yoga. It is important to remember that all practices, whether preliminary or main, have to take place within the sphere of Guru Yoga—uniting with the nature of the guru.

In Guru Yoga, we pray and direct our devotion towards the master who arouses in us the greatest feeling of devotion. Here, we let him appear in the form of the Lotus-born Guru, Guru Rinpoche, who made a solemn promise that for anyone in this degenerate age who has great confidence in him and devotion to him, his blessing would be swifter than that of any other buddha. In his own words:

> Those who accomplish me, accomplish all the buddhas;
> Those who see me, see all the buddhas.

This is his promise, a promise which can never deceive. For although Guru Rinpoche's compassion is the same for all sentient beings, it is particularly swift and powerful for those who live in this decadent age. Reflecting on our own root master, we will see that his qualities have the same nature as those of all the buddhas, and yet his kindness is even greater than theirs because he has come now, at the time when we need him. Take a group of people, for example, who are equally rich; the kindest is the one who uses his or her wealth to help the poor and those who need it most. It is just the same with the master.

If we practice Guru Yoga, perceiving that our root guru is inseparable from Guru Rinpoche, then the blessings we will receive will be both powerful and swift. When an enlightened master who has wisdom and compassion meets a disciple who has faith and diligence, it is as if the sun's rays were suddenly concentrated through a magnifying glass and focused onto dry grass, causing it to burst into flames at once. In the same way, the blessings we receive will correspond directly to the intensity of our devotion.

There are three main parts to the actual practice of Guru Yoga: first there is the visualization, next the fervent prayer to the guru, and lastly the receiving of the four empowerments.

The Visualization

In the sūtras we can read how, on the eve of their attaining enlightenment, bodhisattvas such as Amitābha would make profound prayers and tremendous offerings to all the buddhas. They prayed that they might manifest a buddhafield and then emanate themselves within that buddhafield, so as to bring the greatest possible benefit to all sentient beings.

From the Vajrayāna perspective, however, the understanding of buddhafields is a deeper one. The root of the Vajrayāna is "pure vision," or the perception of the perfect purity of all phenomena. To enact this purity of perception, we do not perceive the place where we are now as just any ordinary place; we imagine it to be a celestial buddhafield. As we recite the description in the visualization, we consider this place itself to be the supreme paradise of Guru Rinpoche, Zangdopalri—the Glorious Copper Colored Mountain—where everything reflects total perfection. The ground is composed of gold, the trees are wish-fulfilling trees, and the rain is the rainfall of nectar. All beings are ḍākas and ḍākinīs; the calls of the birds are the sounds of Dharma; the sounds of nature, wind, water, and fire reverberate as the Vajra Guru mantra; and all thoughts are expressions of wisdom and bliss. So here the perception of purity is much vaster and more omnipresent than in the sūtras.

Within the perfect environment of this self-manifested buddhafield, we visualize ourselves as the mother, or source, of all the buddhas, Vajrayoginī, who is inseparable from Yeshe Tsogyal, the consort of Guru Rinpoche. She is brilliant red, with one face and two hands. In her right hand she wields a hooked knife raised upwards towards the sky, and in her left hand is a skullcup full of blood.[6] In the crook of her left arm is a *khaṭvāṅga* trident, surmounted by a vajra. She stands in a dancing posture on a corpse, a sun disc, and a lotus, poised on her left foot with her right knee bent. She is adorned with the eight bone ornaments: diadem, earrings, three kinds of necklaces, bracelets, anklets, and a bone apron and belt, all encrusted with jewels, and she wears the five silk scarves. Her three eyes gaze in fervent devotion towards the master, Guru Rinpoche.

Her appearance is Yeshe Tsogyal, the consort of the Lotus-born Guru, endowed with all the blessings of the buddhas, while her essence is the manifestation of Jetsün Drölma (Tārā), who carries out the activity of all the buddhas and confers their blessings, benefiting all beings everywhere.

In the sky in front of us or above the crown of our head, seated on the pollen bed of a hundred-thousand-petalled lotus, and a sun and a moon disc, we visualize Guru Rinpoche, the Lotus-born Guru of Oḍḍiyāna, embodiment of all sources of refuge and of the non-dual wisdom of all the buddhas. His nature is that of our root master, the one who has displayed the greatest compassion and kindness towards us, and for whom we have the deepest devotion.

He appears as a beautiful eight-year-old child, his youthful splendor symbolizing his attainment of the unchanging vajra body, which is beyond death. His complexion is white tinged with red, and he is dressed in the robes of the Nine Yānas: a white inner garment underneath, then a blue gown, and upon these the red monastic shawl patterned in gold.

These represent, respectively, the vehicles of the Secret Mantrayāna, the Mahāyāna, and the Hīnayāna. He also wears the monastic skirt, which symbolizes the Śrāvaka and the Pratyekabuddha Yānas, and wrapped around him is a dark blue brocade cape, which represents the Vajrayāna.

He is smiling, with an expression which is at once peaceful and wrathful, indicating his realization of the absolute nature and his subjugation of all negative forces. His eyes gaze straight into the sky; this is the vajra gaze that looks always into the absolute nature. In his right hand he holds a five-pronged golden vajra at the level of his heart. In this degenerate age, however, when evil forces and negative emotions run rampant, we can visualize Guru Rinpoche wielding the vajra in the sky in a gesture of subjugation.

In his left hand, which rests in the mudrā, or gesture, of equanimity, he holds a skullcup that possesses all perfect qualities and characteristics. Within the skullcup is the vase of immortality, overflowing with the nectar of deathlessness. It symbolizes Guru Rinpoche's attainment of the level of vidyādhara of immortality. He sits in the posture of "royal ease," with his right foot slightly extended and his left foot drawn inwards. Just as no one would dare disobey the order of a king, there is no one in the three worlds of saṃsāra who would ever disobey the command of Guru Rinpoche, for he has realized the primordial wisdom of the absolute.

The five buddha-families—buddha, vajra, ratna, padma, and karma—are usually portrayed by their emblems: wheel, vajra, jewel, lotus, and crossed vajras. Here, they are symbolized by Guru Rinpoche's five-petalled lotus crown, which indicates that he belongs to the padma family, and that he is an emanation of Buddha Amitābha. In the crook of his left arm is the khaṭvāṅga trident, representing his secret consort, Mandāravā.

Visualize the Lotus-born Guru clearly, even down to the black and white of his eyes, and the finest details of his clothes. His body is not composed of dense matter like flesh and blood, earth, stone, or gold, but of light, like a rainbow, transparent yet vividly clear. Visualize him there, resplendent amidst an expanse of rainbow light in five colors, which floods the whole of space.

There are three main ways of visualizing Guru Rinpoche and his entourage within this dazzling expanse of light. The first is to visualize all of the gurus of the lineage, from the Primordial Buddha Samantabhadra down to our own root master (in the form of Guru Rinpoche), seated one below the other in a line extending upwards above the crown of our head. The second is to visualize a great gathering, like people in a crowded marketplace, or like massed banks of clouds. The third is to visualize Guru Rinpoche alone as "the one jewel that embodies all," or "the one all-sufficient wish-fulfilling jewel."

Although all three are essentially identical, here we will use the second, and visualize the Lotus-born Guru surrounded by a cloudlike gathering of his retinue. Amongst the retinue are the Eight Vidyādharas of India, holders of the eight transmissions;[7] they include Mañjuśrīmitra, who received the body transmission, Nāgārjuna, who received the speech transmission, and Hūṃchenkara, who received the mind transmission.[8] Also, there are: all of the great siddhas of the New Translation School, such as Drilbupa, who achieved realization through practicing Cakrasaṃvara, and King Indrabodhi, who attained enlightenment through Guhyasamāja; the eighty-four mahāsiddhas of India and those of Tibet; the nine heart-sons and the twenty-five disciples of Guru Rinpoche, as well as the eighty siddhas of Yerpa, who attained the body of light; the hundred and eight great meditators of Chuwori; the thirty mantrikas of Yangzom; the fifty-five *togdens*, or realized beings, of Sheldrak; the twenty-five dākinīs, the seven yoginīs, and many others; the enlightened teachers and saints of the Eight Chariots of Transmission;[9] the great paṇḍitas, accomplished masters and vidyādharas; all the deities of the three roots; the peaceful and wrathful yidams; the ḍākas and ḍākinīs of the three places; the various protectors and guardians of the Dharma; the deities of prosperity; and the protectors of the *terma* treasures.

They fill the sky like a vast cloud and, although they appear as his retinue, as regards their nature there is no distinction between them and Guru Rinpoche, since they are all his emanations. Just as the bodhisattva Norzang attended two hundred and fifty-two spiritual teachers in order to establish auspicious connections, so should we visualize the retinue as a vast gathering in order that we too may be able to meet perfectly enlightened teachers throughout our series of lives. Like the main figure, the deities of the retinue are not substantial like statues; they appear yet they are empty, like reflections of the moon in water. We visualize them as pure and perfect so as to correct and put a stop to our ordinary perception of phenomena as impure. Think of them watching us and smiling with their tremendous compassion, and consider them all as the various aspects of Guru Rinpoche.

This particular teaching of Guru Yoga, as we mentioned earlier, comes from the Longchen Nyingtik, the terma revealed by Jikmé Lingpa. This concludes the first part, the description of the visualization required for accomplishing the practice.

Guru Rinpoche himself made this pledge:

> If you have strong faith and confidence in me,
> I will look on you with compassion: this is my promise,
> And never will I deceive you.

Without this kind of faith and confidence, we cannot receive any blessings, but if we pray to Guru Rinpoche with unfailing confidence and devotion, then there is nothing we cannot accomplish. Being a fully enlightened buddha, he has the power to manifest his wisdom, his loving-kindness, and his strength. And remember that he will never, never desert us, for this was his promise.

Invocation

Having established the visualization, now we invite the wisdom deity from the buddhafields. Just as we would invite an important guest by first preparing our home and then asking him to come, so with the deepest respect we invite Guru Rinpoche with the Seven-Line Prayer, also known as the "Seven Vajra Verses," which is the most essential prayer to Guru Rinpoche.

When the celestial ḍākinīs sang the Seven Vajra Verses, the letter *HRĪḤ*, emanating from the heart of Buddha Amitābha, descended upon a red lotus blossom on the Lake of Milk[10] in the northwest of the land of Oḍḍiyāna, and transformed into an eight-year-old child—Guru Rinpoche, the Lotus-born. Later, at the time when Guru Rinpoche was meditating in the Eight Great Cemeteries, the ḍākas and ḍākinīs sang this Seven-Line Prayer to invite him and to request him to turn the Wheel of Dharma.

The Seven-Line Prayer carries the essence of all Guru Rinpoche's blessings. As Guru Rinpoche said: "To this very prayer, you can give your whole mind, in devotion." He also said:

> When a disciple calls upon me with yearning devotion,
> And with the sweet-sounding song of the Seven-Line
> Prayer,

> I shall come straightaway from Zangdopalri,
> Like a mother who cannot resist the call of her child.

The Seven-Line Prayer is to be found in all of the teachings of Guru Rinpoche revealed by the hundred and eight major and one thousand minor *tertöns,* or treasure-discoverers. So it is a prayer that is most extraordinary, easy to practice, and replete with immense blessings.

To invoke the Lotus-born Guru, we recite the Seven-Line Prayer three times. At the same time, in the sky before us, we visualize the paradise of Zangdopalri with Guru Rinpoche and his retinue of vidyādharas, ḍākas, and ḍākinīs. Then, what we visualize in the sky dissolves into the visualization we have already created. The buddhafield dissolves into the buddhafield, Vajrayoginī dissolves into Vajrayoginī, Guru Rinpoche dissolves into Guru Rinpoche, and the retinue of deities, ḍākas, and ḍākinīs into the corresponding retinue. In this way, the *jñānasattva,* the wisdom deities invited from the buddhafields, and the *samayasattva,* which is our initial visualization, merge indivisibly into one.

Do not ever think that the buddhafields are far away, or doubt whether the buddhas may or may not come. For as Guru Rinpoche said:

> I am present in front of anyone who has faith in me,
> Just as the moon casts its reflection, effortlessly, in any vessel filled with water.

The Seven Branches of Devotional Practice

So as to receive Guru Rinpoche's blessings, we also need to complete the accumulation of merit and wisdom. The easiest and, at the same time, the most essential method for this is the one in seven branches. Praised by all the sages of the past, these seven branches condense all the many different ways of accumulating merit.

(1) Prostration

The first of the seven branches is to pay homage with prostrations. When we accomplish the preliminary practices of Ngöndro, we perform 100,000 prostrations either while reciting the refuge formula during the refuge practice, or while reciting the seven branches of devotional practice during Guru Yoga. In the same way that someone becomes very humble when they are in front of a person who commands great respect, our humility should increase when we do this practice in the presence of Guru Rinpoche and all the buddhas.

Visualizing ourselves in our ordinary form, we put aside all arrogance and pride, and demonstrate our respect by offering prostrations. There are three ways of performing prostrations. The highest is with the View, while recognizing the absolute nature—the essence of buddhahood. The next is through meditation, where we visualize ourselves in an infinite number of forms, all prostrating in unison towards the source of refuge, and all reciting the prayer in seven branches, as if we were leading the prayers of all sentient beings. The third kind is where we generate faith and devotion as we prostrate ourselves on the ground towards the source of refuge.

To do prostrations properly, you touch the ground with five points—the forehead, the two hands, and the two knees. Another method, used by the Kadampas, is to fling yourself forward, letting the hands hit the ground before the knees. This is known as the full or extended prostration and is the most secret way of purifying impairments of the samaya.

Before we begin the prostration, first we join the palms of our hands together at the level of our heart. The hands should not be held pressed flat against each other, but with an empty space in between them, so that they resemble a lotus bud about to burst into bloom. This symbolizes the blossoming of our bodhicitta. Then we raise our two joined hands to our forehead, consider that we are prostrating to the body aspect of all the buddhas, and pray:

> May all the obscurations of my body be dispelled and
> May I receive the blessing of realizing the body of all the buddhas!

Then we place our hands at the level of the throat, consider that we are prostrating to the speech aspect of all the buddhas, and pray:

> May all the obscurations of my speech be purified and
> May I receive the blessing of realizing the speech of all the buddhas!

Finally, we place our hands at the level of our heart and pay homage to the heart, or mind, aspect of all the buddhas, praying:

> May all the obscurations of my mind be clarified and
> May I receive the blessing of realizing the mind of all the buddhas!

Then we prostrate and consider that when the five points touch the ground the five poisons are purified into the five wisdoms.

The benefits of doing prostrations are inconceivable. As it says in the sūtras:

> The number of particles of dust beneath your body when doing just a single prostration to the Lord Buddha will be the number of times you will be reborn as a universal monarch in future lives.

(2) Offering

Offering includes both material offerings and offerings visualized by the mind. For the material offerings, we offer as much as we can, particularly the seven traditional offerings: water, flowers, incense, lamps, scented water, food, and music. For the offerings visualized by the mind, we imagine mountains, forests, beautiful plants, gardens, oceans, and all the ornaments and precious things of the universe and its inhabitants. We also visualize that the whole sky is filled with the eight auspicious signs and the eight auspicious ingredients,[11] along with beautiful jewels, palaces, and celestial gardens.

All of this is offered without the slightest expectation of any reward, as an antidote to greed and miserliness. Then we consider that out of their compassion and wisdom the buddhas joyfully accept our offering, so that we can accumulate merit.

(3) Confession

We use confession to purify our negative actions, our defects and downfalls, for if such stains are not purified they will create a barrier to realization. In order to purify negative actions, obscurations, and defilements, we need to rely upon four strengths, namely: the strength of the support, the strength of regret, the strength of the antidote, and the strength of the promise.

The first is the strength of the support. Just as when a criminal appears in a court of law, the judge is surrounded by all those who represent justice, so too when we visualize Guru Rinpoche above our head, he is surrounded by a retinue of buddhas, bodhisattvas, and vidyādharas. This is the object to whom we present our regret and confession.

The second is the strength of regret. If we had not committed any negative actions in the past, there would be nothing to confess and nothing to repair. So we acknowledge how throughout our countless lives we have repeatedly committed transgressions against the three vows: the pratimoksha vows, the bodhisattva vows, and the commitments of the Secret Mantrayāna. If these are not purified, they become like a poison inside us, and are responsible for our continuing to wander in saṃsāra.

Third is the strength of the antidote, which is the actual practice of purification. With ardent devotion, we pray to Guru Rinpoche and imagine that boundless rays of light stream out from his heart center and dissolve into us. This light cleanses us completely, as it washes out and dissolves all our imperfections and negativities. Finally Guru Rinpoche, with a radiant smile, says to us: "All of your obscurations are purified."

Lastly there is the strength of the promise, which means to make an unshakable resolution: "From now on—even if my life is at stake—I shall never again indulge in negative actions."

With these four strengths, all our negative actions can be purified. As it is said: "Negativity does have one good quality—it can be purified."

(4) Rejoicing

Whenever we think of the good accumulated by others, however great or small, and we rejoice sincerely, from our hearts and without a trace of jealousy, this mere act of rejoicing will cause us to accumulate the same merit as if we had carried out those positive actions ourselves. Think about how Guru Rinpoche manifested in this universe: he came, free from any of the stains of the obscuring emotions, and benefited beings in all the three worlds through his countless emanations, turning the Wheel of Dharma and teaching the Nine Yānas. If we rejoice wholeheartedly at such wonderful deeds, then we actually share in their merit. The same holds true whenever we experience a deeply felt joy at any virtuous action performed by others—teachers, disciples, hermits, or anyone who benefits others. So this rejoicing should be sincere, and come from the depths of our hearts.

(5) Requesting the Turning of the Wheel of Dharma

Of all the activities of a buddha in bringing benefit to beings, the most precious and the most fundamental is turning the wheel of the three vehicles of the Dharma. After attaining enlightenment, Buddha Śākyamuni remained silent for three weeks to emphasize the rarity and value of the teachings. Then Brahmā and Indra came from their celestial kingdoms to request the Buddha to turn the Wheel of Dharma for the good of all beings. Brahmā offered him a thousand-spoked golden wheel and Indra offered a white conch shell that coiled to the right. As a result of their request, the Lord Buddha first turned the Wheel of Dharma in the Deer Park at Vārāṇasī, when he taught the Four Noble Truths. He then turned the Wheel of Dharma a second time at the Vulture Peak, where he gave the teachings on emptiness, and a third time in various places, when he unfolded the ultimate truth of the union of emptiness and manifestation.

In the same way, if we request the teacher to turn the Wheel of Dharma according to the different needs and capacities of beings, then we will share in that merit. And as a result, we are rendering a great service to the teachings and to the Dharma as a whole.

(6) Requesting the Buddhas and Teachers to Remain

The teachings given by enlightened beings are the expression of their inner realization, which is why we should request the buddhas and masters not to pass away into nirvāṇa, but to remain until saṃsāra has been emptied. Realized beings who have attained the bodhisattva levels are not subject to ordinary birth and death, and when their activity is complete, they dissolve their physical form altogether. This is why we need to request them, as fervently as possible, to remain longer, in order to help all sentient beings, and to bring them to the level of buddhahood.

(7) The Dedication of Merit

What we dedicate now includes the merit of offering this prayer in seven branches, as well as all the merit we have accumulated in the past or will accumulate in our future lives. The way in which we dedicate this merit is limitless, emulating the buddhas and bodhisattvas of the past when they shared and distributed their merit among all sentient beings, and free from clinging to the three saṃsāric concepts of an actor, an action, and an object of action. This implies that we have completely realized the view of emptiness, but even if we have not, whenever we dedicate, it should be free from any ordinary clinging.

Devotion and Blessing

Devotion is the heart of the Guru Yoga practice; in fact it is the very practice itself. The qualities of devotion are respect, yearning, and ardent faith. Without devotion, the seed of liberation will shrivel and die, whereas with devotion all the noble qualities of the path to enlightenment will blossom and grow.

As beginners, we may well find that our faith and devotion are not spontaneous, and so at first it is important to generate that feeling actively, over and over again. To do this, we call to mind the qualities of the guru, especially his kindness in leading us out of saṃsāra, and in granting us his profound instructions. To help us remember that kindness, we visualize him above the crown of our head and pray to him with intense devotion. As a result, our contrived devotion will gradually be transformed into a spontaneous and continuous one. Devotion will become so much a part of our stream of thought that at the mere mention or recollection of the guru's name, all ordinary perceptions will stop, disturbing emotions will no longer arise, and our thoughts will constantly flow towards the master. This means that our mind will remember nothing but the teacher; it will be completely captivated by him.

Then whatever good fortune may come our way, such as an increase in wealth, fame, or favorable conditions, we will realize that this is due to the kindness of the master. Yet we will also know that all these achievements are like a dream, devoid of any essence, and so we will be free from any pride or clinging. We will be glad, for example, to use all this dream-like wealth as an offering to the guru.

On the other hand, if all kinds of undesirable circumstances and difficulties befall us, or people criticize us, we will understand this as the fruit of having harmed others during our previous lives. Thinking of how we can purify our karma through this suffering, we pray to the guru: "May you grant me your blessing so that I can purify my past actions, and may my suffering completely exhaust the suffering of all other beings." And so we will come to view unfortunate circumstances as an expression of the guru's activity, there to help us purify our obscurations.

By thinking only of the guru, a fervent devotion will arise, and our eyes will fill with tears. As Guru Rinpoche said:

> Complete devotion brings complete blessing;
> Absence of doubts brings complete success.

It is through a devotion such as this that the realization of wisdom will blossom within us. All the noble qualities of the Nine Vehicles, from the vehicle of the Śrāvakas up to the unsurpassed Dzogpachenpo, are all born from the blessings of the guru. So devotion should be recognized as the principal seed, the source, for progressing along the path, for dispelling obstacles and ultimately for attaining enlightenment.

This part of the Guru Yoga opens with a prayer[12] to the Lotus-born Guru which begins with the words: "Jetsün Guru Rinpoche…," meaning, "O Guru Rinpoche, Precious One…"

If we pray with the deepest fervor, and with a prayer as ardent and moving as this, then the blessings will swiftly enter our being. When we say, "Jetsün," it indicates that Guru Rinpoche is the principal presence among all the buddhas and deities, and that he is the lord of all maṇḍalas. The word "guru" literally means one who is "weighty," and implies that the guru is someone replete with all the qualities of buddhahood. "Rinpoche" means "great jewel." Such a jewel has six qualities: it is rare, flawless, powerful, supreme, unchanging, and the ornament of the universe.

Consider that, outwardly, the guru is the union of the Three Jewels: his body is the Saṅgha, his speech the Dharma, and his mind the Buddha. Inwardly, he embodies the three roots: his body is the lama (guru), his speech the yidam (deva), and his mind the khandro (ḍākinī). Secretly, the guru is the union of the three kāyas: his body is the nirmāṇakāya, his speech the sambhogakāya, and his mind the dharmakāya. The guru is also the union of all deities, for there is not a single deity who is not the display of the Lotus-born Guru. In the unsurpassable buddhafield of Akaniṣṭha, he is the Primordial Buddha Samantabhadra. He is also Vajradhara, or Dorje Chang. In the sambhogakāya buddhafields, he is Vajrasattva and the buddhas of the five families. In the nirmāṇakāya buddhafields, he is the Buddha Śākyamuni and the Lotus-born Guru, Padmasambhava. In brief, there is no manifestation of the Buddha that is not inseparably one with Guru Rinpoche, and so to pray to him is the same as praying to all the buddhas.

If we can pray with real fervor to Guru Rinpoche, he will remove all obstacles and enable us to progress along the path. All buddhas have the same compassion and the same love for sentient beings, but Guru Rinpoche has for countless *kalpas*[13] made powerful prayers to benefit the beings of this difficult, decadent age, who are the victims of so much torment. If we pray fervently to him, he will look on us as his only child, and he will come at once, from the land of the *rākṣasas* in the southwest, to appear before us.

Whenever we pray to Guru Rinpoche, we should not just mouth the words, but pray one-pointedly from the core of our heart, from the marrow of our bones, and with a devotion that consumes our mind.

To attain the omniscient state of buddhahood, it is necessary to realize the empty nature of all phenomena, through which the wisdom inherent in our fundamental buddha nature is unveiled. In the Root Vehicle of Characteristics, it takes three great kalpas of accumulating merit to achieve such realization. But through the path of devotion to the teacher, even an ordinary individual will achieve realization in one lifetime, thanks to the power of devotion and the blessings of the guru. On the other hand, to expect realization without faith and devotion is the same as hoping that the sun will rise on a cave that faces north.

We should constantly keep in mind that Guru Rinpoche is our sole refuge, whether in happiness or in sorrow, whether in the higher realms of saṃsāra or the lower. Without any second thoughts, we should give our whole mind to him, like throwing a pebble into a lake.

The era in which we now live is known as the "Age of Five Degenerations." Our lifespan is shorter than it was in the Golden Age; this is the degeneration of life. Also, it is very rare to find someone who practices the Dharma and whose behavior really accords with it; this is the degeneration of karma, or activity. This world of ours is constantly stricken by wars, famine, and disease, and there is but little hope of peace and happiness; this is the degeneration of the times. All the while, the root causes of this general degeneration are the intense emotions that plague beings: hatred, desire, misjudgment, pride, and envy; this is the degeneration linked with emotions. Finally, beings even turn their back on the Dharma; this is the degeneration of the view.

We have to wake up to the desperate and miserable conditions of this age; instead of finding it a source of fascination and pleasure, we ought to feel like a fish writhing on a hook. We need to turn to Guru Rinpoche, the perfect buddha who vowed especially to help the beings of these decadent times, and call out to him with ardor and with longing: "There is no other hope for me but you! Unless you take me under your protection, I shall sink even deeper into saṃsāra's ocean of suffering." This is how the sun of Guru Rinpoche's compassion, concentrated now through the magnifying glass of our devotion, will set fire to the dry grass of our ignorance and destructive emotions.

The Vajra Guru Mantra

Although at present we do not have the good fortune to see Guru Rinpoche's face or to hear his voice, we have his mantra, which he blessed with his wisdom, loving-kindness, and strength to be identical with him. This mantra is not composed of ordinary syllables, but has the power to dispel all obstacles and confer all the qualities of wisdom.

The scriptures tell us there is no mantra that carries more benefit than the Vajra Guru mantra. Its twelve syllables are the essence of the twelve branches of Lord Buddha's teachings.[14] Bearing in mind the inconceivable benefit of reading the whole Tripiṭaka, if the twelve-syllable mantra is its essence, we can begin to appreciate the sheer power of its blessings. Then, our ceaseless wandering in saṃsāra is due to the interplay of the Twelve Links of Interdependent Origination, which arise from ignorance and culminate in our taking rebirth over and over again.[15] By reciting the twelve-syllable mantra, these twelve interdependent links are purified, releasing us at last from saṃsāra. The Vajra Guru mantra can be explained in many ways, and in particular in terms of nine levels related to the Nine Vehicles. Such explanations can be found in a terma revealed by Karma Lingpa, in the writings of Dodrupchen Jikmé Tenpé Nyima, and in other scriptures.

OṂ ĀḤ HŪṂ

The first three syllables of the mantra represent the three kāyas, as well as the vajra body, speech, and mind of all the buddhas. *OṂ* corresponds to the dharmakāya, the nature of Buddha Amitābha; *ĀḤ* corresponds to the sambhogakāya, and the Lord of Compassion, Avalokiteśvara; *HŪṂ* corresponds to the nirmāṇakāya, manifesting as the Lotus-born Guru, Padmasambhava.

VAJRA

The vajra (*dorje* in Tibetan) refers to the diamond, the hardest and most precious of all stones. A diamond can cut through all other substances, yet cannot itself be cut by any of them. This symbolizes the unchanging, non-dual wisdom of the buddhas, which cannot be affected or destroyed by ignorance, but cuts right through all delusions and obscurations. It indicates too that the qualities and activities of the body, speech, and mind of the buddhas can benefit all sentient beings, without hindrance from negative forces. Like a diamond, the vajra is free from all defects. Its indestructible strength comes from the realization of the dharmakāya nature, the nature of Buddha Amitābha.

GURU

As we have seen, the word "guru" in Sanskrit means "weighty," or "heavy." Just as gold is the heaviest and most precious of metals, the guru is the most weighty and most precious of all beings, because of his inconceivable and flawless qualities. Here the guru corresponds, on the sambhogakāya level, to Avalokiteśvara, who is endowed with the seven branches of union.[16]

PADMA

Padma, meaning "lotus" in Sanskrit, indicates the padma family from the five buddha-families. These five families—buddha, vajra, ratna, padma, and karma—are represented by the five buddhas: Vairocana, Akṣobhya, Ratnasambhava, Amitābha, and Amoghasiddhi, respectively. Guru Rinpoche is the nirmāṇakāya emanation of Amitābha, who corresponds to the lotus family and the speech aspect of the buddhas. It is stated in the sūtras that simply by uttering the name of Buddha Amitābha, you will be reborn in Sukhāvatī, the Paradise of Great Bliss, never to be reborn again in lower realms. In the same way, reciting the name of the Lotus-born Guru will bring us every kind of realization.

The incomparable qualities of the six-syllable mantra, the *Maṇi*, are also described in all the scriptures as being able to bring us to the realization of the bodhisattva levels, or *bhūmis*. The Maṇi mantra of Avalokiteśvara is the sambhogakāya aspect of the Vajra Guru mantra, and also corresponds to the great Vairocana Buddha.[17] This buddha, who is the size of the whole universe, holds a begging bowl in his two hands in the mudrā of equanimity. It is said that within this begging bowl is a lotus with twenty-five rows of petals arranged one upon the other. These rows correspond to the various aspects of the body, speech, mind, qualities, and activity of the buddhas. For example, the body alone has five subdivisions: body-body, body-speech, body-mind, body-qualities, and body-activity. The present nirmāṇakāya paradise of the Buddha Śākyamuni is said to rest at the level of the heart, and corresponds to the row of the mind-mind subdivision, this being the reason why in this paradise the precious teachings of the Secret Mantrayāna—the Vajrayāna—could be taught and spread.

SIDDHI

The word *siddhi* means "true accomplishment." By remembering and praying to the body, speech, mind, qualities, and activity of Guru Rinpoche, both ordinary and supreme accomplishments will be ours. Ordinary accomplishments include freedom from sickness and endowments such as wealth and prosperity; the supreme accomplishment is to attain the complete realization of Guru Rinpoche himself.

HŪṂ

Reciting the syllable *HŪṂ* is like requesting or invoking the guru to come and to bless us with all the siddhis, ordinary and supreme.

Our master, Guru Rinpoche, and the mantra are inseparable. So when we utter the name of the guru by reciting the mantra, it's as if we are calling out repeatedly to someone who simply cannot fail to reply. The guru cannot but turn his compassion towards us, and so, if we pray one-pointedly like this, there is absolutely no doubt that Guru Rinpoche will come at once to grant us his blessings. When rain falls on the earth, it falls evenly everywhere, but only the good seeds will germinate, not the rotten ones. In the same manner, the compassion of Guru Rinpoche is unbiased; it is directed universally to all beings, and yet his blessings will be swifter for those who have devotion and faith.

It is only through the blessings of a buddha that we can achieve realization. So a prayer like this, one that invokes Guru Rinpoche's very name, must go out from the marrow of our bones, from the core of our heart; then gradually our devotion will become spontaneous and unceasing. Remember that without faith, there will be no accomplishment. At the time of the Lord Buddha, for example, there were those who could see and hear him in person, and still had no faith in him.[18] Some of the heretical teachers even tried to poison him. Similarly, when Guru Rinpoche went to Tibet, the evil ministers plotted and schemed to kill him. For people such as these, spiritual accomplishment is out of the question.

This shows how important it is to have a faith that is very pure and genuine. And so, as a support, we visualize our outer environment as Zangdopalri, the beings around us as ḍākas and ḍākinīs, ourselves as Yeshe Tsogyal, and above our head Guru Rinpoche, surrounded by his retinue. Then we pray, reciting the prayer in seven branches and the other prayers in the practice, with the confidence and trust that by so doing, accomplishment will surely blossom.

The Lineage Prayer

The Dzogchen teachings are transmitted in three ways: from mind to mind, by signs, and through oral transmission.[19]

In the first, the mind-to-mind transmission, there is no need for symbols or words, as the teacher and the retinue are by their very nature one. This is the way in which the transmission was given from the Primordial Buddha Samantabhadra to Vajrasattva, and from him to Garab Dorje.[20]

After Garab Dorje, the transmission continued with Mañjuśrīmitra, Śri Siṁha, Jñānasūtra, and Vimalamitra. Although these masters manifested in human form, there was no need for them to give or receive transmission by words, since they were all fully realized beings. The transmission was effected simply by "signs"—by mudrās or by symbolic utterances. When the master gives transmission in this way, the disciples apprehend its meaning at once and achieve complete realization of the three categories of Dzogpachenpo: mind, space, and pith instructions.

The oral transmission was passed from one individual to another, beginning with Guru Rinpoche. He gave it to his disciples: the twenty-five main disciples, the eighty siddhas of Yerpa, the fifty-five realized beings of Sheldrak, and others.

Guru Rinpoche's three main disciples were King Trisong Detsen, Vairocana, and his consort Yeshe Tsogyal. The transmission then continued up until the Omniscient Longchen Rabjam, from whom it passed to the great Vidyādhara Jikmé Lingpa, who transmitted these profound treasures to his disciples. His four principal disciples were called "the four Jikmés,"—"the four fearless ones." Of these four, the two main ones were Dodrupchen Jikmé Trinlé Özer and Jikmé Gyalwé Nyugu, an emanation of Avalokiteśvara; the two others were Jikmé Gocha and Jikmé Ngotsar. From Jikmé Trinlé Özer the transmission went to the great siddha Do Khyentse Yeshe Dorje, and from Jikmé Gyalwé Nyugu it passed to Jamyang Khyentse Wangpo; both Do Khyentse and Jamyang Khyentse Wangpo were authentic emanations of Jikmé Lingpa. The two lineages then fused in the great teachers Gyalsé Shenpen Tayé, Patrul Rinpoche, and Khenpo Pema Dorje. They in turn transmitted it to Wönpo Tenga, Nyoshul Lungtok, Adzom Drukpa, the third Dodrupchen Jikmé Tenpé Nyima, and many other masters. Again, these lineages came together in the person of Jamyang Khyentse Chökyi Lodrö, who was the emanation of Jamyang Khyentse Wangpo.[21]

This is how this lineage of individuals has remained unbroken down to the present day. Although we say "individuals," they are all realized beings who dwell in the bhūmis, the levels of the bodhisattvas. Now, so that we can receive the blessings of these gurus, we need to pray to them with one-pointed devotion.

The Practice of Dzogpachenpo

As for the practice of these teachings, there are several methods, which correspond to the capacity of the individual.

Ordinary individuals simply endeavor to discriminate between what is to be done and what is to be avoided, with the goal of attaining the temporary happiness of this life.

Individuals of *medium* capacity will recognize that the very nature of the three worlds of cyclic existence is suffering, and by reflecting on this, they will realize the preciousness of this human body, which is the support for attaining enlightenment. They will contemplate impermanence, which is the spur to their diligence, without ever forgetting that death may come at any time. Then they will realize how it is their own actions that are the cause of either suffering or happiness. Having seen that suffering pervades saṃsāra entirely, a strong feeling of renunciation and of wanting, by every means possible, to free themselves from saṃsāra will arise in their minds.

Yet the wish to free ourselves from this ocean of suffering is not enough on its own; as we have seen, we need to rely upon a guide, an object of refuge. Supreme amongst them all is the vajra master, the authentic teacher qualified with all the signs of an accomplished being. Once we have found such a teacher, we need to protect our spiritual link with him as carefully as we would protect our very eyes.

To do this, we need to be wise in three different ways. First, we should be wise in finding an authentic teacher and examining his qualities through learning about his life and his teachings. Then, when we have found a teacher, we should be wise in attending to him perfectly, following his instructions to the letter. Finally we should be wise in realizing his instructions, by practicing them. If we are wise in these three ways, then we will travel along the path without effort and without error.

There are also three levels of pleasing the guru and fulfilling his wishes. The best is to achieve the supreme accomplishment of enlightenment through the practice—to realize the View through meditation and action. The next best is to serve the teacher with your body, speech, and mind. The third is to make material offerings towards his work and teachings.

We progress along the Mahāyāna path by taking refuge and generating the enlightened mind of bodhicitta. Then, in order to dispel the obscurations and negative actions which create hindrances on the path, we perform the purification practice of Vajrasattva, and in order to gather favorable conditions through accumulating merit, we make the maṇḍala offering. Finally we arrive at the Guru Yoga practice, the most essential practice for awakening and arousing wisdom.

The aim behind each and every one of these practices is not merely to meditate, to perform certain activities, or to recite a large number of prayers. They are all different means towards succeeding in our main purpose, which is to train and transform our mind. As it is said:

> Transform your mind, and you will be perfect;
> All bliss comes from taming the mind.

So make a firm resolution, and decide: "From now until I die I will practice diligently, all of the time." If we can do so, we will end up like Jetsün Milarepa, who accomplished the greatest method of pleasing the guru: attaining enlightenment. Since the very reason the guru has come into this world is to show us the path, the best way to fulfill his wishes is to realize the teachings. But as Jikmé Lingpa pointed out: "Theory is like a patch, one day it will just wear off." We need to integrate the teachings into our experience, and make them an intrinsic part of our being, otherwise they are not really of much use.

Finally, for beings of *superior* capacity, there are the profound paths of the development or generation stage (Mahāyoga), the completion stage (Anuyoga), and then the most sublime path of all, the Dzogpachenpo (Atiyoga).

Mahāyoga

Having met a precious teacher, been accepted by him, and received his profound instructions, now we come to put the instructions into practice. To do so, we need to transform our impure perception of outer phenomena into a vision of infinite purity.

To practice the inner tantra, we need to realize that *everything* is primordially pure. Accordingly, the outer elements are not perceived as ordinary, but as the five female buddhas. The five aggregates within the body are also not perceived as ordinary, but as the five male buddhas. In the same way, the eight conciousnesses as well as their eight objects are perceived as the eight male and eight female bodhisattvas. Through this kind of perception, not only do we come to see the purity of all phenomena, but also we will perceive the "great evenness of saṃsāra and nirvāṇa." No longer then will we look upon saṃsāra as something to be discarded and nirvāṇa as something to be attained; they will be seen and understood as the "union of great purity and great evenness." Yet a state like this is not something which has to be fabricated anew; it has always been there, since the very beginning.

The essence of Kyérim—the development, or generation stage—or Mahāyoga, is to recognize all appearances as the deity, all sounds as mantra, and all thoughts as the dharmakāya. This is the most profound path, through which we can actualize all of the qualities of the body, speech, and mind of the Buddha. We say "actualize," because these are but the expression of the primordial nature of things, which is now simply being revealed.

Anuyoga

The practice of the completion stage, or Anuyoga, is based mainly upon the Six Yogas: *tummo*, or inner heat, the root of the path; *gyulü*, or illusory body, the foundation of the path; *milam*, or dream, the measure of progress along the path; *ösel*, or luminosity, the essence of the path; *bardo*, or the intermediate state, the invitation to continue on the path; and *phowa*, or transference of consciousness, which will allow us to travel the remainder of the path.

Atiyoga

The practice of Dzogchen or Atiyoga is to realize the *tathāgatagarbha*, or "buddha nature," which has been present as our true nature since the very beginning. Here it is not sufficient to focus on contrived practices that involve intellectual effort and concepts. To recognize our true nature, the practice should be utterly beyond fabrication. The practice is simply to realize the emptiness and the radiance, or natural expression, of wisdom, which is beyond all intellectual concepts. It is the true realization of the absolute nature just as it is—the ultimate fruition.

At the moment, our awareness—rigpa—is entangled within our mind, completely enveloped and obscured by mental activity. Through the practice of Trekchö, or "cutting through all attachment," and the "direct realization" of Tögal, we can unmask this awareness and let its radiance arise.

To accomplish this, we need to practice "the four ways of leaving things in their natural simplicity" (*chokshyak*) and by means of them, to acquire perfect stability in the Trekchö practice. Then will come the "four visions of Tögal," which are the natural arising of visions of discs and rays of light, deities, and buddhafields. These visions are naturally ready to arise from within the central channel that joins the heart to the eyes. This arising from the central channel will appear in a gradual process: in the same way that the waxing moon increases from the first to the fifteenth of the month, these visions will gradually increase—from the simple perception of dots of light to the full array of the vast expanse of the sambhogakāya buddhafields. The manifestation of space and awareness will thus reach its culminating point.

These experiences are not linked with consciousness or intellect as former experiences were; they are a true manifestation, or radiance of awareness. After this, in the same way that the moon decreases and disappears from the fifteenth to the thirtieth of the month, all of these experiences and visions—all phenomena—will gradually come to exhaustion and reabsorb themselves in the absolute. At this point the deluded mind which conceives subject and object will disappear, and the primal wisdom, which is beyond intellect, will gradually expand. Eventually you will attain the perfect enlightenment of the Primordial Buddha Samantabhadra, endowed with the six extraordinary features.[22]

This is the path intended for people of superior faculties who can achieve enlightenment in this very lifetime. For those of *medium* capacity, there is the instruction on how to achieve liberation in the bardo, or intermediate state. When we say "bardo," in fact we recognize four bardos: the bardo from conception until death, the bardo of the moment of death, the bardo of the absolute nature, and the bardo of coming into the next existence.[23]

The bardo between conception and death is our present state. In order to destroy all deluded perceptions or deluded thoughts in this bardo, the ultimate practice is Dzogchen Atiyoga, in which there are the two main paths of Trekchö and Tögal, as described above. The ultimate fruition of this practice comes when the ordinary body made of gross aggregates dissolves into the "rainbow body of great transference," or "vajra body," or it dissolves without leaving any physical remains.

But even if we cannot achieve such ultimate attainment within one lifetime, there is still the possibility of achieving enlightenment at the time of death. If our teacher or a close Dharma brother or sister is near us at the very moment of our death, he or she will remind us of the instructions—the introduction to the nature of mind. If we can recall our experience of practice and remain in this nature of mind, we will achieve realization. It is then possible to depart to a buddhafield straightaway with no intermediate state. If this is not accomplished, then the bardo of the absolute nature, or *dharmatā,* will arise. At this point, the ground luminosity of the dharmakāya will appear. If we can unite the ground luminosity, or "mother luminosity," with the luminosity that we have recognized while practicing during our lifetime, called the "child luminosity," then we will be liberated into the dharmakāya.

If we are not liberated at this time, then countless manifestations will appear, of sounds, lights, and rays. Tremendous fear will strike us because of these emanations and visions, but if we are good practitioners, we will realize that there is no point in being afraid. We will know that whatever deities appear, wrathful or peaceful, they are all our very own projections. To recognize this is to ensure liberation in a sambhogakāya buddhafield.

But if this is not accomplished, then the bardo of coming into a new existence will ensue. This is when, if we practice in the right way, we can be liberated into a nirmāṇakāya buddhafield.

Essentially, the primordial nature of the Buddha Samantabhadra is like the ground or mother-nature of realization. The nature which has been introduced to us by the teacher is like the child-nature. When these two meet, we will attain complete realization and seize the fortress of enlightenment.

Even *ordinary* beings, unable to achieve liberation either in this life or in the intermediate state, can attain it in the nirmāṇakāya buddhafields.

To summarize then, through the practice of the path of Trekchö and Tögal we can reach the ultimate realization of the dharmakāya, the enlightened state of the Primordial Buddha Samantabhadra, within this very lifetime. This is in the best case. If not, then we can be freed in the other three bardos: the bardos of the moment of death, of dharmatā, and of rebirth. Even if this does not happen, we can still be relieved of suffering and be liberated through the virtues or blessings of the Dzogchen teachings. Whoever has a connection with them is: liberated by sight, on seeing the teaching or the teacher; liberated by hearing, on hearing the teacher or teaching; liberated by contact, on wearing the precious mantras and scriptures of Dzogpachenpo; or liberated by taste, and so on. As a result, we will be liberated into one of the five nirmāṇakāya buddhafields, that of Vairocana, Akṣobhya, Ratnasambhava, Amitābha, or Amoghasiddhi, and finally into the central buddhafield—"the Cemetery of the Blazing Mountain."[24]

The Four Empowerments

With the skillful means of the Vajrayāna, the practitioner receives the blessings of the teacher in the form of rays of light. This is the empowerment (*abhiṣeka* in Sanskrit, or *wang* in Tibetan). It is called "empowerment" because when we receive it we are empowered to follow a particular spiritual practice, and so come to master its realization. Most of us have received empowerment from a qualified teacher, but to maintain the stream of blessings of the empowerment and to renew its power, we need to receive the four empowerments over and over again by ourselves, through the practice of Guru Yoga. This is in fact the most essential part of the Guru Yoga practice.[25] In Guru Rinpoche's own words:

> If you received an empowerment every year and lived for a hundred years, it would add up to one hundred empowerments. Then, even if you had to be reborn among the animals, it would be as their king.

The empowerment is the most essential way to receive the blessings of the guru's body, speech, mind, and wisdom, which will dispel the veils and obscurations of our own body, speech, mind, and inherent wisdom.

In order for us actually to receive these four empowerments, first of all we fervently invoke the gurus of the lineage with the Lineage Prayer, at the end of which all the lineage masters, yidams, ḍākas, and ḍākinīs melt into light and dissolve into our root teacher, whom we visualize above our head in the form of Guru Rinpoche. Now he becomes even more radiant and even more resplendent than before, as within him are gathered the compassion and wisdom of all the buddhas of past, present, and future.

The Vase Empowerment

Brilliant rays of white light, radiating like the "water-crystal moon," stream out from a white syllable *OṂ* at Guru Rinpoche's forehead center. They are absorbed into a white letter *OṂ* visualized in our own forehead center, and completely fill our entire body—we are still visualizing ourselves as Vajrayoginī. Through this, all the stains and obscurations due to negative actions of our body are dispelled,[26] and our channels (*nāḍī* in Sanskrit, *tsa* in Tibetan) are purified.

Within our body, we have three main channels, but because of our ignorance and delusion, it is karmic energy (inner air or "wind") that circulates through these channels. They are blocked by twenty-two knots that bind the two lateral veins to the central one and prevent the circulation of wisdom energy, thereby creating deluded perceptions. As these knots untie, two by two, we reach the levels of realization from the first to the eleventh bhūmi, which is buddhahood.

Through receiving the blessing of the body of the guru in this first empowerment, all of the obscurations, stains, and impurities of the channels are purified. We receive the Vase Empowerment, which empowers us to meditate upon the development stage, or Kyérim—in other words, to meditate upon a deity. We might ask: What is the point of meditating upon deities? This kind of meditation allows us to realize that all appearances *are* primordially pure: the universe *is* a buddhafield and all beings *are* ḍākas and ḍākinīs, manifestations of the guru; all sounds *are* the natural resonance of mantras; and all thoughts *are* the movements of wisdom. In our present state, we are deceived by appearances, so that whenever we see beautiful forms, we are attracted by them, and when we see ugly forms, we are repelled or disgusted. This is the very cause of our wandering in saṃsāra.

Through the practice of Kyérim, pure perception will arise, and this is a sign that delusion has been dispelled. In truth, what is simply being revealed is the natural state of things, for example, that the five elements *are* the female buddhas of the five families, and the five aggregates *are* the male buddhas of the five families.

Through receiving the first empowerment, the seed for attaining the level of the completely matured vidyādhara, or "wisdom-holder," is sown within us.[27] At this level the mind of the practitioner has been transformed, or matured, into wisdom. Although his body is still there as an envelope, it is not made of ordinary aggregates, and is ready to dissolve into the wisdom body at the moment of death. In the same way that a fish placed on dry ground can be quite sure it will not survive for very long, the yogin whose mind has been freed into wisdom knows that this is his last ordinary body, and that as soon as this corporeal envelope is destroyed at death, he will achieve liberation. The level of the completely matured vidyādhara corresponds to the path of accumulation and the path of preparation in the five paths of the Sutrayāna teachings.[28] Through this empowerment the seed for realizing the nirmāṇakāya is sown within our being.

The Secret Empowerment

The second empowerment, which confers the blessing of the guru's speech, is known as the Secret Empowerment. From a red syllable *ĀḤ* at the throat center of the guru stream out boundless rays of brilliant ruby-colored red light. These are absorbed into a syllable *ĀḤ* visualized at our own throat center, and they completely fill our whole body. This purifies the four negative actions committed through speech: lies, divisive talk, harsh words, and irrelevant chatter.

There are three constituents to our body: the channels, energy, and essence. The channels were purified by the first empowerment; in the second empowerment the karmic energy (or wind: *prāṇa* in Sanskrit, *lung* in Tibetan), which gives rise to attachment, hatred, and all ordinary deluded thoughts and actions, is purified into wisdom energy. This karmic energy is like a blind horse carrying the crippled rider of the mind here, there, and everywhere. Since energy and mind are so closely related, by purifying the karmic energy into wisdom, the deluded mind is purified into primordial awareness. So when the red light pervades our body and all its channels, the wisdom of bliss-emptiness dawns in our being and we receive the second empowerment.

The Secret Empowerment empowers us to practice the recitation of mantras. We might ask: Why are mantras so important? It is because they are not mere words or ordinary sounds; they have been blessed by the deity to be the same as the deity itself. Mantras also include the name of the deity, so just as when you call someone over and over again they cannot help but reply, the deities cannot fail to bless us.

Of the four vidyādhara levels, the second empowerment will bring the realization of the vidyādhara who has power over life. The name itself shows that such a being has realized the unchanging nature of the absolute, and that both body and mind have been transmuted into wisdom.

Of the four kāyas, this empowerment sows the seed for realizing the sambhogakāya, within which is found the display of the five celestial buddhafields, located in the center and the four cardinal directions.

The Wisdom Empowerment

This is the empowerment of the heart, or mind, of the guru and is known as the Wisdom Empowerment. At Guru Rinpoche's heart center is a syllable *HŪṂ*, clear blue like an autumn sky, which sends out boundless rays of dazzling blue light. They dissolve into another blue syllable *HŪṂ* visualized in our own heart center, and completely fill our whole body. With this, the three defects or negative actions of mind—covetousness, malice, and wrong views—are purified, and we receive the blessings of the guru's mind, the non-dual wisdom of all the buddhas.

Of the three constituents of the body, here the essence (*bindu* in Sanskrit, *tiklé* in Tibetan), which is carried along the channels by the energy, is purified. There are both red and white tiklés, which in ordinary states are the cause of the various experiences of bliss and suffering. When these are purified, all the obscurations of the mind as well as the latent tendencies are purified, giving birth to absolute wisdom.

We are empowered to practice the various concentrations of Śamatha (*shyiné* in Tibetan), or "tranquil abiding," and Vipaśyanā (*lhaktong* in Tibetan), or "greater vision," through which we can recognize the true nature of the guru.

In fact, that which is to be realized, the nature of emptiness, has no substance, color, or shape, and recognition of this comes about when we experience the Great Bliss of Wisdom. This is an all-pervading bliss that has nothing to do with ordinary, deluded bliss. Great Bliss is generated through the practice of tummo. In this practice, the practitioner visualizes, below the navel center, a point resembling the right stroke of the Tibetan letter *A*. From it rises fire, swift and strong, which ascends through the channels to a white syllable *HAṂ* visualized at the top of the head. Touched by the fire, the *HAṂ* begins to drip a precious nectar, which fills the practitioner's body with an experience of Great Bliss, unstained by ordinary emotions.

Through the Wisdom Empowerment, of the four vidyādhara levels we will here attain that of the mahāmudrā vidyādhara. When Guru Rinpoche granted the empowerment of Vajrakīlaya to his disciples, he assumed the form of Vajrakīlaya at the center of the maṇḍala. Such a capacity to display an infinite number of wisdom forms is the fruit, or characteristic, of this vidyādhara level. It demonstrates that body, speech, and mind are now pervaded with wisdom.

Of the four kāyas, with this empowerment we establish an auspicious connection for realizing the dharmakāya, which is the pure dimension of the mind.

The Symbolic Empowerment

The fourth empowerment is known as the Ultimate Empowerment of the Absolute Nature. The blue syllable *HŪṂ* at the guru's heart center emanates another syllable *HŪṂ* which, like a shooting star, flies into our heart, instantly filling our whole body with light. All the subtle defilements that mask realization are purified, and deluded perceptions, dualistic clinging to subject and object, as well as all latent tendencies, are dispelled. The subtle defilements upon the universal ground (*kunshyi* in Tibetan) are purified. The universal ground is where the residue of past actions, our habits and tendencies, which create obstacles on the path to enlightenment, are stored. According to the Sutrayāna, the subtle obscurations that veil realization are only cleared when we reach the tenth bhūmi. However, according to the Secret Mantrayāna, when our own awareness is seen as immaculate and becomes as vast as the sky, all the subtle defilements veiling the knowable are dissolved.

Now all the subtle stains caused by the ten unvirtuous actions of body, speech, and mind are purified, particularly the defilements concealing the "vajra wisdom." Here, vajra wisdom refers to the inseparability of the enlightened body, speech, and mind of the guru. For although on a relative level we may distinguish between the vajra body, speech, and mind, in reality they are all aspects of one nature, known as vajra wisdom. The body of a buddha is uncompounded, like the sky; his speech is the source of the eighty-four thousand sections of the Dharma; and his mind is sheer awareness. Yet these three are indivisible, and any one of the body, speech, or mind of a buddha can express the qualities of the other two.

This empowerment is called the Symbolic Empowerment because it indicates the absolute wisdom. Yet a mere indication is not wisdom itself, because words cannot describe the absolute. Through the blessing of such an empowerment—the transference of the guru's blessings—we will actually realize this wisdom for ourselves.

With this empowerment, we are empowered to meditate on Dzogpachenpo and we will reach the level of the spontaneously accomplished vidyādhara, which is equivalent to the level of buddhahood, and the indivisibility of the three kāyas—the svābhāvikakāya.

Through the blessing of the guru, our body, speech, and mind and the guru's enlightened body, speech, and mind will become indistinguishably one. Here, we simply remain in equipoise, within the state of emptiness and pure awareness.

At the end of the practice, we arouse an even stronger devotion towards the master, as a result of which the guru becomes even more resplendent in compassion and kindness, and smiles at us with tremendous love. Then a red light streams out from his heart like a shooting star, is absorbed into our heart, and fills our whole body with inconceivable bliss. As we experience this bliss, our body melts into a mass of red light the size of an egg, which gradually condenses into an exceedingly brilliant red sphere. Like a spark of fire, it suddenly shoots out and dissolves into Guru Rinpoche's heart. We then remain in this state, our mind inseparable from the wisdom mind of Guru Rinpoche.[29]

Ordinarily speaking, the mind is that which constantly remembers different thoughts and actions, negative and positive, happy or sad. Yet if we examine this mind, we find that past thoughts are now completely gone; they are dead, like a corpse. Future thoughts are not yet born—we have no idea what will come into our mind tonight. So past and future thoughts do not exist. Then, if we also look into the present thought, we will see that even that does not exist; there is nothing, in fact, but emptiness.

So, just remain in a state of recognition, a fresh and vivid simplicity, the nature of the guru, in which our mind is not inferior in comparison with his, but all is merged into one nature. We should remain in this natural state for as long and as often as we can.

The Essence of Guru Yoga

When thoughts arise, we imagine ourselves once more as Vajrayoginī, with Guru Rinpoche above our head. There is no need to do an elaborate visualization of the retinue and all the other details. Simply maintaining the presence of the guru above our head, we carry a strong feeling of devotion throughout all our daily activities.

The essence of Guru Yoga is simply to remember the guru at all times: when you are happy, think of the guru; when you are sad, think of the guru; when you meet favorable circumstances, be grateful to the guru; and when you meet obstacles, pray to the guru, and rely on him alone. When you are sitting, think of the guru above your head. When you are walking, imagine that he is above your right shoulder, as if you were circumambulating him. When you are eating food, visualize the guru at your throat center and offer him the first portion. Whenever you wear new clothes, first offer them to the guru, and then wear them as if he had given them back to you.

At night, when you are about to fall asleep, visualize Guru Rinpoche in your heart center, the size of the first joint of your thumb, sitting on a four-petalled red lotus. He is emanating countless rays of light, which fill your whole environment, melting the room and the entire universe into light, and then returning to absorb into your heart. Then the guru himself dissolves into light. This is the state in which you should fall asleep, retaining the experience of luminosity. If you do not fall asleep, you can repeat the visualization again.

When you wake up in the morning, imagine that the guru emerges from your heart and rises up to sit again in the sky above your head, smiling compassionately, amidst a mass of rainbow light.

This is how we can remember the guru and apply devotion during every activity. And should death come suddenly, the best practice then is to blend our mind with the mind of the guru. Of all the sufferings of the three intermediate states, the most intense is the suffering of the moment of death. For this moment there are practices of Phowa, or the transference of consciousness to the buddhafields. The practice of Guru Yoga is the most profound and essential way of doing Phowa.

Finally, this practice of Guru Yoga is sealed with a profound prayer:

> May I and all sentient beings reach the ultimate goal of the path: the realization of the absolute nature!
> Having obtained this human body, met the teacher, received his instructions, and put them into practice,
> May we make the seeds of the four empowerments blossom into the four kāyas, so dispelling the four veils!
> By accomplishing the four kāyas, may we achieve ultimate enlightenment!

It is with this wish-fulfilling prayer and many others like it that we should put the ultimate seal on all our practice.

In brief, and to conclude, Guru Yoga is the essence of all practices and the easiest on which to meditate. It entails no danger and it is endowed with boundless blessings. It has been the main object of practice of all the enlightened beings of India and Tibet, and in all the different schools. Through the Guru Yoga practice, all obstacles can be removed and all blessings received. And through merging our mind with the mind of the guru, and remaining in the state of inseparable union, the absolute nature will be realized. This is why we should always treasure Guru Yoga and keep it as our foremost practice.

In general, as I mentioned at the beginning, any practice or activity that we undertake must be governed by the Three Noble Principles. The first is to practice not for ourselves alone, but for all sentient beings, and therefore we generate the most precious attitude—that of wishing to guide all beings to the state of enlightenment.

Second, the main part of the practice is to practice one-pointedly as we go through each step of the preliminary practice: the four thoughts, refuge and bodhicitta, the Vajrasattva practice, the maṇḍala offering, and Guru Yoga. Actions performed with the body, recitation of the speech, and concentration of the mind should all be done one-pointedly and without distraction. While we concentrate on what we are doing with the body, we must not let our speech drift into ordinary conversation. When we recite with our mouth, we must not let our mind wander away from the practice. The main part of the practice then is to be single-mindedly focused and to be free from any clinging, so that the benefit of our practice will not be carried away by outer circumstances. For more advanced practitioners this second point means to dwell constantly in the realization of the emptiness of all phenomena.

The third Noble Principle is to conclude by dedicating the merit of the practice. Whatever merits we may have accumulated in the past, and may accumulate in the future, we dedicate to all sentient beings so that they may achieve buddhahood. Our aspiration when we dedicate should have the same expansive and generous attitude as that with which the vast merit of the buddhas and bodhisattvas is dedicated.

Conclusion

This particular Guru Yoga practice belongs to the tradition of the Longchen Nyingtik. However, this does not mean that it is in any way limited because it belongs to one particular lineage. Although here we find Guru Rinpoche at the center of the practice, and in the new translation traditions the Buddha Vajradhara, or Dorje Chang is the central figure in the Guru Yoga, they are identical in nature. The main point is to practice the Ngöndro preliminary practice in a genuine way. It is *the* prerequisite for having a sound foundation for the main practice. Without the Ngöndro, the main practice will not resist deluded thoughts, it will be carried away by circumstances, it will be unstable, and it will not reach its ultimate goal. It will be like building a beautiful mansion on a frozen lake. No main practice should start without the foundation of the preliminary practice. And as it says in the concluding verses of this text by Jikmé Lingpa:

> Through accomplishing this preliminary practice, you will eventually be reborn in the paradise of Zangdopalri, the Glorious Copper Colored Mountain.

So, at present you may be living in a country distant from the land where the Buddha's teaching was born, yet thanks to your good fortune you have been able to meet the Dharma and start practicing. This is a sign that you have a good connection. But in order to progress along the path you need to find a qualified teacher, otherwise all your efforts will be wasted. Having found a teacher, you should then practice in accordance with his instructions, remembering that within the preliminary practice all the vital points of the paths of sūtra and tantra are included, and that you are truly fortunate to be able to practice them.

I received these teachings many times from my teacher Jamyang Khyentse Chökyi Lodrö, as well as from Shechen Gyaltsap Rinpoche, and now I have shared the essence of them with you.

The Guru Yoga Practice

from the Preliminary Practice of Longchen Nyingtik[30]

The Visualization

Emaho!

My entire perception, spontaneously perfect, is a realm of infinite purity,

The Glorious Copper Colored Mountain, arrayed in complete and perfect detail. Here, in its very center,

My own body is Vajrayoginī,

With one face and two hands, brilliant red and holding hooked knife and skull,[31]

My two feet gracefully poised, my three eyes gazing into the sky.

Above my head, on a blossoming hundred-thousand-petalled lotus, sun- and moon-disc seat,

Inseparable from my own root master, embodiment of all sources of refuge, appears

Guru Rinpoche, in the supreme nirmāṇakāya form of the "Lake-born Vajra."

His body glows with youth, white with a tinge of red.

He wears a gown, monastic shawl, cloak and robe,

With one face, two hands, and in royal poise.
In his right hand he holds the vajra, in his left a skullcup containing the vase of immortality,
On his head he wears the five-petalled lotus hat,
Cradled in his left arm he holds the "supreme consort" of bliss and emptiness,
Concealed as the three-pointed khaṭvāṅga trident.
He presides amidst a shimmering aura of rays and rings of rainbow light.
All around him, enveloped in a beautiful lattice of white, blue, yellow, red, and green light,
Are King Trisong Detsen, the twenty-five disciples,
The paṇḍits, siddhas, and vidyādharas of India and Tibet, yidam deities,
Ḍākinīs, and dharmapālas and protectors who keep the samaya—all gather like billowing clouds,
Visualized vivid and distinct, in the great equality of clarity and emptiness.

The Seven-Line Prayer

Hūṃ!
In the northwest of the land of Oḍḍiyāna,
In the heart of a lotus flower,
Endowed with the most marvelous attainments,
You are renowned as the "Lotus-born,"
Surrounded by hosts of ḍākinīs.
Following in your footsteps,
I pray to you: Come, inspire me with your blessing!
GURU PADMA SIDDHI HŪM

The Seven Branches of Devotional Practice[32]

Prostration

Hrīḥ!
As many times as there are atoms in the universe,
I multiply my body and offer you prostrations.

Offering

With both real offerings and those created in the mind
through the power of samādhi,
I offer the entire universe in one vast gesture of offering.

Confession

All the harmful actions of my body, speech, and mind,
I confess and purify in the luminosity of dharmakāya.

Rejoicing

Whether they be relative or absolute,
I rejoice in all positive, virtuous actions.

Requesting the Turning of the Wheel of Dharma

According to the receptivity and needs of different beings,[33]
I implore you to turn the Wheel of Dharma of the Three
Yānas.

Requesting the Buddhas and Teachers to Remain

Till saṃsāra is completely empty, and all beings liberated,
Do not pass into nirvāṇa, but remain here among us, I pray.

The Dedication of Merit

All the merit and positive actions of past, present, and
future,
I dedicate so that all beings may attain supreme
enlightenment.

Maturing the Siddhi

O Guru Rinpoche, Precious One,
You are the embodiment of
The compassion and blessing of all the buddhas,
The only protector of beings.
My body, my possessions, my heart and soul

Without hesitation, I surrender to you!
From now until I attain enlightenment,
In happiness or sorrow, in circumstances good or bad, in situations high or low,
I rely on you completely, O Padmasambhava, you know me: think of me, inspire me, guide me, make me one with you!

OṂ ĀḤ HŪṂ VAJRA GURU PADMA SIDDHI HŪṂ

Invoking the Blessing

I have no one else to turn to;
In these evil times, the beings of the Kaliyuga
Are sinking in a swamp of intense and unbearable suffering.
Free us from all this, O Great guru!
Grant us the four empowerments, O blessed one!
Direct your realization into our minds, O compassionate one!
Purify our emotional and cognitive obscurations, O powerful one!

OṂ ĀḤ HŪṂ VAJRA GURU PADMA SIDDHI HŪṂ

I pray to you from the bottom of my heart,
It's not just words or empty mouthings:
Grant your blessings from the depth of your wisdom mind,
And cause all my good aspirations to be fulfilled, I pray!

OṂ ĀḤ HŪṂ VAJRA GURU PADMA SIDDHI HŪṂ

The Lineage Prayer

Emaho!
In the heavenly realm, free from all dimensions and extremes,
Is the Primordial Buddha, the dharmakāya Samantabhadra;[34]

His wisdom-play, like the reflection of the moon in water,
the sambhogakāya Vajrasattva;
Perfect with all buddha-qualities, nirmāṇakāya
Garab Dorje;
To you I pray: Grant me your blessings and empowerment!

Śri Siṁha, treasure of the ultimate Dharma;
Mañjuśrīmitra, universal ruler of the Nine Yānas;
Jñānasūtra, great paṇḍita Vimalamitra:
To you I pray: Show me the way to make my mind free!

Padmasambhava, sole ornament of this world of ours,
Your supreme heart-disciples, Trisong Detsen, Vairocana,
Yeshe Tsogyal, and the rest;
The one who revealed a vast ocean of wisdom mind
treasures, Longchenpa;
Entrusted with the space treasury of the ḍākinīs, Jikmé
Lingpa:
To you I pray: Grant me liberation and fruition!

Master of the Dharma, Changchub Dorje;
The siddha, Jikmé Gyalwé Nyugu;
Supreme among emanations, Mingyur Namkhé Dorje;
Son of the buddhas, Shenpen Tayé;
To you I pray: Show me my original face!

Glorious heruka, Do Khyentse Yeshe Dorje;
Patrul Rinpoche, Orgyen Jikmé Chökyi Wangpo;
Lord of siddhas, Padma Vajra;
Padmasambhava himself, great Khyentse Wangpo;
To you I pray: Grant me siddhis, ordinary and supreme!

Natsok Rangdrol, who self-liberated all the dharmas of
saṃsāra and nirvāṇa;[35]
Omniscient Jikmé Tenpé Nyima;
Embodiment of all sources of refuge, Chökyi-Lodrö:
To you I pray: Bless my mind, inspire my understanding!

Prayer for This Life

Through true renunciation and disgust for saṃsāra,
May I rely upon my vajra-lama meaningfully, as though he were my very eyes,
Following his instructions to the letter, and taking to heart the profound practices he gives,
Not just now and then, but with diligent and constant application,
May I become worthy of the transmission of his profound wisdom mind!

Since all appearances, saṃsāra and nirvāṇa, from the very beginning are the Akaniṣṭha pure realm of the buddhas,
Where all perception is liberated into perfect buddha forms, all sounds are purified into mantra, all thoughts are matured into dharmakāya reality,
And since Dzogpachenpo is free of any effort of abandoning and adopting,
And since rigpa's self-radiance is beyond thoughts and experience,
May I see the naked reality of dharmatā!
May all ordinary clinging to reality be totally liberated into rainbow light,
And the experiences of kāyas and tiklés increase!
May rigpa's strength be enhanced, maturing into the fullness of sambhogakāya perfection!
As all perception of phenomenal reality wears out, and the conceptual mind dies into the state of total enlightenment,
May I gain the stronghold of the Youthful Vase body, free from birth and death!

Prayer for the Bardo

But if I am not able to master the practice of the great Atiyoga in this life,
And this gross physical body is not liberated into the pure space of the rainbow body,

Then when the constituents of life itself fall apart,
At the moment of death may the ground luminosity arise as the dharmakāya, pure from the beginning;
May appearances of the bardo experience be liberated into sambhogakāya forms;
And, perfecting the path of Trekchö and Tögal,
May I be liberated, as naturally as a child running into its mother's lap!

Prayer for the Next Life

In this great Secret Mantrayāna path of luminosity—Dzogpachenpo—the summit of all,
Enlightenment is to be sought nowhere but in the face of the dharmakāya:
If I am not liberated into the primordial state by actualizing this,
Then, through perfecting the five practices of "enlightenment without meditation,"[36]
May I be born into the nirmāṇakāya realms of the five buddha-families,[37]
And especially in the "Palace of Lotus Light," the Zangdopalri heaven of Guru Rinpoche,
In the presence of the Lord of Orgyen himself, chief of the ocean of vidyādhara masters,
While he is celebrating the feast of the great Secret Mantra Dharma,
Let me be born as his favorite son or daughter,
To take upon myself the task of helping limitless beings!

Prayer of Fulfillment

Through the inspiration and blessing of the ocean of victorious vidyādharas,
By the truth of the infinite Dharmadhātu, beyond conception,
And with this free and well-favored human form, may I enact the interconnectedness of

Perfecting the qualities of the buddhas, ripening sentient beings, and purifying realms,
And attain the state of buddhahood!

Receiving the Four Empowerments

The Vase Empowerment

In the Guru's[38] forehead is the letter *OṂ*, radiant and shimmering like moonlight;
From it rays of light stream out and enter my forehead.
Negative actions of the body and blockages of the channels[39] are purified.
The blessing of the vajra body of the buddhas enters me,
The Vase Empowerment is obtained,
I become a receptive vessel for the visualization practice of Kyérim,
The seed of the completely matured vidyādhara is sown.
The potential of obtaining the level of nirmāṇakāya is implanted within me.

The Secret Empowerment

In his throat is the letter *ĀḤ*, blazing like a ruby;
From it rays of light stream out and enter my throat.
Negative activity of the speech and blockages of the inner air[40] are purified,
The blessing of the vajra speech of the buddhas enters me,
The Secret Empowerment is obtained,
I become a receptive vessel for mantra recitation practice,
The seed of the vidyādhara with power over life is sown.
The potential of obtaining the level of sambhogakāya is implanted within me.

The Transcendent Knowledge-Wisdom Empowerment

At his heart, from the letter *HŪṂ*, sky-colored rays of light stream out
And enter my heart.

Negative activity of the mind and blockages of the energy[41] are purified.
The blessing of the vajra mind of all the buddhas enters me,
The Transcendent Knowledge-Wisdom Empowerment is obtained,
I become a receptive vessel for the Caṇḍāli practice of bliss and emptiness,
The seed of the mahāmudrā vidyādhara is sown.
The potential of obtaining the level of dharmakāya is implanted within me.

The Word or Symbolic Empowerment

Again, from *HŪṂ* in his heart, a second letter *HŪṂ* bursts out like a shooting star
And merges, indistinguishably, one with my own mind.
The karma of the "ground of all"[42] and cognitive obscurations are purified,
The blessing of the vajra wisdom enters me,
The empowerment of the absolute truth, symbolized by the Word, is obtained.
I become a receptive vessel for Dzogpachenpo, pure from the very beginning,
The seed of the spontaneously accomplished vidyādhara is sown.
The potential of the svābhāvikakāya—the final fruition—is implanted within me.

OṂ ĀḤ HŪṂ VAJRA GURU PADMA SIDDHI HŪṂ[43]

The Dissolution

When my life is at an end,
With my entire perception the heaven of Ngayab Ling, the Glorious Copper Colored Mountain,
The nirmāṇakāya pure land of indivisible appearance and emptiness,
My body, Vajrayoginī,

Is transformed into a radiant, shimmering sphere of light
And, merging, totally inseparable from Padmasambhava,
I will attain buddhahood.
Then, from the play of vast primordial wisdom,
Which is the miraculous manifestation of bliss and emptiness,
For every single being in the three realms,
Let me appear as their true guide, to lead them to liberation—
Jetsün Padma, grant this, I pray!

From the heart-center of the Lama a beam of light, red and warm, suddenly bursts out and touches my heart; till now I visualize myself clearly as Vajrayoginī. Instantaneously I am transformed into a sphere of red light the size of a pea, which shoots up towards Padmasambhava, like a spark that spits from the fire. It dissolves into Guru Rinpoche's heart, merges and becomes one with him: one taste.

Concluding Prayers

Glorious Tsawé Lama, precious one,
Dwell on the lotus-seat in the depth of my heart,
Look upon me with the grace of your great compassion,
Grant me the attainments of body, speech, and mind!

Towards the lifestyle and activity of the lama,
May wrong view not enter in for even a moment, and
May I see whatever he does as a teaching for me:
Through such devotion, may his blessing infuse and
inspire my mind!

In all my lives, may I never be separated from the perfect Lama;
May I enjoy the complete benefit of the Dharma,
And so perfect the qualities of the five paths and ten stages,
And swiftly attain the sublime level of Vajradhara!

Long Life Prayer for Dilgo Khyentse II of Shechen, Urgyen Tenzin Jigme Lhundrup

Composed by Kyabjé Trulshik Rinpoche

Oṃ Svasti!
Through the compasion of infinite buddhas and bodhisattvas,
And the blessing of wondrous gurus, devas, and ḍākinīs,
The beloved master Khyentse, treasure of knowledge and love,
Has manifested his matchless emanation, just as all have wished:
Fearless Holder of the Teachings of the Lord of Orgyen
And of the nonpartisan tradition of sūtras and tantras,
All victorious one, let your life be forever firm and indestructible:
And accomplish, spontaneously and without effort, your vision—of present happiness and ultimate bliss!

♦ ♦ ♦

For the sake of auspiciousness, our guide throughout saṃsāric existence and the peace of nirvāṇa, our refuge and protector, the supreme lord of victorious ones, His Holiness the Dalai Lama, kindly bestowed a name upon the precious reincarnation of the lord of refuges, the great Vajradhara Dilgo Khyentse, at the long life cave of Māratika, at the same time as he was offered a set of robes. There, on the excellent eighth day of the waxing phase of the auspicious eleventh month of the Wood Pig year—Friday, 29 December 1995—the bewildered bhikṣu Shadeu Trulshik, Vāgindra Dharmamati, wrote and offered this, with a single-minded aspiration. Jayantu!

Acknowledgments

Our deepest thanks go to Shechen Rabjam Rinpoche, Dzongsar Khyentse Rinpoche, Dzigar Kongtrul Rinpoche, and Tsikey Chokling Rinpoche for contributing the foreword and preface. Mention must be made here of the great debt of gratitude owed by so many to Pema Wangyal Rinpoche, who brought Kyabjé Dilgo Khyentse Rinpoche and numerous other great masters to the West, and made their teachings available to Western practitioners.

We would like to thank Könchog Tenzin, Matthieu Ricard, for all the care and attention he gave both to the translation and to *Guru Yoga* in general. Special thanks also to Jeff Cox, Chris Hatchell, and all at Snow Lion Publications, as well as to those members of Rigpa who took part in the editing process.

Patrick Gaffney
Rigpa International

Notes

1. Matthieu Ricard, *Journey to Enlightenment: The Life and World of Khyentse Rinpoche, Spiritual Teacher from Tibet* (New York: Aperture, 1996), pp. 7-8.

2. For the biography of Jikmé Lingpa and the revelation of the Longchen Nyingtik, see Tulku Thondup, *Masters of Meditation and Miracles* (Boston: Shambhala, 1996), pp. 122-128, Janet Gyatso, *Apparitions of the Self* (Princeton University Press, 1988), and Dilgo Khyentse, *The Wish Fulfilling Jewel* (Boston: Shambhala, 1988), pp. 4-8.

3. Eight freedoms and ten advantages constitute a precious human birth. The eight unfavorable conditions to be free from are: birth in hell, hungry ghost, or animal realms, amongst the gods or barbarians or those who have wrong views, in an age where no buddha has come, or without all one's faculties intact. Of the ten favorable conditions, five are intrinsic: to be born a human being, in a land where Dharma can be found, with faculties intact, without a negative lifestyle, and having faith in the Three Jewels. Five are external: the Buddha has come, he has taught the Dharma, it has survived, it is practiced, and we are guided by a spiritual teacher.

4. Śrāvakas and Pratyekabuddhas, the "listeners" and "those who become buddhas by themselves," form the Saṅgha, or community, of the Hīnayāna (or Fundamental Yāna). Dilgo Khyentse, *The Wish-Fulfilling Jewel* (Boston: Shambhala, 1988), p. 105.

5. For example, in the Longchen Nyingtik the outer method is this Guru Yoga practice, "The Wish-fulfilling Jewel," the inner method is the sādhana of Guru Rinpoche, "The Assembly of the Vidyādharas—Rigdzin Düpa," the secret practice is where Guru Rinpoche appears in the form of Avalokiteśvara, "The Self-liberation of Suffering—Dukngel Rangdrol," and the innermost secret practice focuses on Longchenpa with the Primordial Buddha Samantabhadra in his heart, "The Sealed Quintessence—Tiklé Gyachen."

6. Patrul Rinpoche, in *The Words of My Perfect Teacher* (San Francisco: HarperCollins, 1994), p. 313, says: "With her right hand she is playing a small skull-drum held up in the air, awakening beings from the sleep of ignorance. Her left hand is resting on her hip, holding the curved knife that cuts the root of the three poisons." When the visualization emphasizes Yeshe Tsogyal, she is described as above, whereas if the emphasis is on Vajrayoginī, she is described in her usual form, holding a hooked knife and skullcup filled with *amṛta*, or blood.

7. These are the Eight Sādhana Teachings (Drubpa Kagyé) on the eight herukas, or chief yidam deities, of Mahāyoga, transmitted to the Eight Great Vidyādharas.

8. Of the Eight Great Vidyādharas, Mañjuśrīmitra was the holder of the transmission of the body aspect of the yidam Yamāntaka—the wrathful form of Mañjuśrī. Nāgārjuna received the speech aspect, Hayagrīva, and Hūṃkara (or Hūṃchenkara) the mind aspect, Viśuddha (Yangdak Heruka).

9. The Eight Chariots of Transmission, or great practice lineages which thrived in Tibet, are: Nyingma, Kadam, Sakya, Marpa Kagyü, Shangpa Kagyü, Shyijé and Chö, Jordruk (Kalachakra: Dorje Naljor), and Dorje Nyendrup (or Orgyen Nyengyü).

10. The Dhanakośa Lake in northwest Oḍḍiyāna; in Sanskrit, *dhana* means "wealth" and *kośa* "treasury."

11. The eight auspicious signs, or symbols, are: the parasol, golden fishes, treasure vase, lotus flower, right-turning conch shell, glorious endless knot, banner of victory, and wheel. The eight auspicious ingredients, or objects, are: mirror, *ghiwang* medicine, yoghurt, *durva* grass, *bilva* fruit, right-turning conch shell, cinnabar, and mustard seeds.

12. See p. 77.

13. A kalpa is a vast period of time corresponding to the life-cycle of a universe, including its formation, duration, destruction, and the interim period that follows. See Dilgo Khyentse, *The Heart Treasure of the Enlightened Ones* (Boston: Shambhala, 1992), p. 218.

14. The twelve branches of Buddha's teaching are: general discourses (sūtras), teachings through song, prophecies, verse, teachings to maintain the Dharma, teachings after specific incidents, anecdotes, stories of the past, previous lives, extremely detailed teachings, wondrous teachings, and establishing the meaning of the teachings through classification, description, and enumeration.

15. The Twelve Links of (Inter)dependent origination are: ignorance, karmic propensities, conditioned consciousness, name and form, the six sense fields (the five senses and mind), contact (sense impressions), feeling, desire or craving, grasping and attachment, coming into being (existence), birth, and old age and death.

16. The seven branches of union of the sambhogakāya, or seven aspects of supreme union, are explained by Dilgo Khyentse Rinpoche:

> Whatever manifestations of realms, palaces and forms there are, peaceful and wrathful deities, they do not exist on a gross level. They are forms of shunyata endowed with all the supreme qualities. Therefore, they are known as possessing the aspect of being without self-nature.
>
> The minds of those buddhas are completely filled with the wisdom of unchanging non-dual bliss-emptiness. Therefore, they are known as possessing the aspect of union.
>
> Their body, speech, and mind are eternally filled with the taste of great bliss, free from increase and decrease. Therefore, they are known as possessing the aspect of great bliss.
>
> In the realm and palace, none of the chief and retinue, devas and devis, have ever known suffering. They are completely endowed with all the good qualities of saṃsāra and nirvāṇa. Therefore they are known as possessing the aspect of complete enjoyment.
>
> Their wisdom of great bliss is free from meditation and postmeditation, neither increases nor decreases, and is without change or cessation. Therefore, they are known as possessing the aspect of freedom from interruption.
>
> As for themselves, they achieved such virtues, but through compassion, they eternally care for confused sentient beings. Therefore, they are known as possessing the aspect of having a mind completely filled with great compassion.
>
> Their buddha activity tames others at all times in all directions throughout the three times. Therefore, they are known as possessing the aspect of continuity.

Quoted in Nalanda Translation Committee, *The Rain of Wisdom* (Boston: Shambhala, 1980), pp. 341-342.

17. See Jamgön Kongtrul Lodrö Tayé, *Myriad Worlds* (Ithaca: Snow Lion, 1995), pp. 98-104.

18. "The monk Sunakshatra was the Buddha's half brother. He served him for twenty-four years, and knew by heart all the twelve categories of teachings in the pitakas. But he saw everything that the Buddha did as deceitful, and eventually came to the erroneous conclusion that, apart from an aura six feet wide, there was no difference between the Buddha and him... Because he did not have the slightest faith and held only wrong views, (he) ended up being reborn as a *preta* (a hungry ghost) in a flower garden." Patrul Rinpoche, *The Words of My Perfect Teacher* (San Francisco: HarperCollins, 1994), pp. 147, 21.

19. The three transmissions are: the Mind Direct Transmission of the Buddhas, the Sign Transmission of the Vidyādharas, and the Oral Transmission of Realized Beings.

20. For the lives of all the lineage masters mentioned here, see Tulku Thondup, *Masters of Meditation and Miracles* (Boston: Shambhala, 1996).

21. Kyabjé Dorjechang Jamyang Khyentse Chökyi Lodrö (1896-1959) was the activity emanation of Jamyang Khyentse Wangpo, and the teacher of Kyabjé Dilgo Khyentse Rinpoche.

22. The six extraordinary features of the liberation of Samantabhadra are:

1. This liberation arises to our own awareness as the display of this awareness. There are no deluded perceptions that come from clinging to this display as an outer phenomenon.
2. This liberation transcends the aspects of "primordial ground" and "manifestation that arises from the primordial ground." If not, there would be a possibility of falling into delusion as phenomena arise from the primordial ground.
3. If we recognize the primordial wisdom free from all obscurations, at that very instant all the qualities that dwell naturally within the expanse of that wisdom spontaneously appear. We realize that the obscurations related to the various karmic tendencies accumulated upon the amorphous basic consciousness are pure from the very beginning. Like a brilliant sun emerging from the clouds, we transcend utterly the ground of saṃsāra.
4. At the same instant, transcendent insight matures as the kāya of the ultimate nature itself; we conquer the citadel of primordial purity and dwell there immutably.
5. The actualization of our own awareness is not born from outer circumstances provided by something other than awareness

itself, and it is independent of all conditions. Buddhahood is achieved through awareness recognizing its own nature, through its own strength.

6. The ground for liberation dwells primordially in the continuum of its own nature, and cannot be penetrated by the causes of delusion.

23. Also known as the natural bardo of this life, the painful bardo of dying, the luminous bardo of dharmatā, and the karmic bardo of becoming. See: Sogyal Rinpoche, *The Tibetan Book of Living and Dying* (San Francisco: Harper, 1992), and Tsele Natsok Rangdröl, *The Mirror of Mindfulness* (Boston: Shambhala, 1989).

24. The central buddhafield, "Cemetery of the Blazing Mountain," is the central buddhafield of the maṇḍalas of the wrathful deities. According to the higher tantras of the Nyingma tradition, to enter this buddhafield corresponds to ultimate enlightenment.

25. See "Receiving the Four Empowerments of Ngöndro Practice" in Tulku Thondup, *Enlightened Journey* (Boston: Shambhala, 1995), pp. 191-230.

26. The three harmful physical actions are: taking life, taking what is not given, and sexual misconduct.

27. Or "knowledge holder with residues," see Tulku Thondup, *Enlightened Journey,* pp. 218-220.

28. The five paths are the paths of accumulation, preparation, seeing, meditation, and no more learning.

29. This is also the practice of phowa, the transference of consciousness at the moment of death.

30. The arrangement of the Guru Yoga here is as practiced in the tradition of Jamyang Khyentse Chökyi Lodrö. The translation of the Guru Yoga practice is in part by Sogyal Rinpoche and in part by Rigpa Translations.

31. See note 6, above.

32. The seven branches serve as antidotes: prostration is the antidote to pride; offering is the antidote to attachment, greed, meanness, and poverty; confession is the antidote to aggression and anger; rejoicing is the antidote to envy and jealousy; requesting the turning of the Wheel of Dharma is the antidote to ignorance; requesting the buddhas and teachers to remain is an antidote to wrong views; and dedication is an antidote to uncertainty and doubts.

33. This line was composed and added by Jamyang Khyentse Wangpo. The Tibetan actually reads "For disciples of the three kinds...." These three kinds of capacity, ability, or receptivity can refer to either the Śrāvakas, Pratyekabuddhas, and bodhisattvas, or to the three scopes or kinds of individuals.

34. From Samantabhadra to Vajrasattva is considered as the Mind Direct Lineage of the Buddhas; from Garab Dorje to Padmasambhava, the Sign Lineage of the Vidyādharas; and from then on the Oral Lineage of Realized Beings.

35. Adzom Drukpa (1842-1924).

36. Liberation through: seeing cakras, hearing mantras and dhāraṇīs, tasting nectar, touching the mudrā, and remembering the phowa.

37. The five pure realms are: Ngönpar Gawa (Vajra-East); Paldangdenpa (Ratna-South); Pema Tsekpa (Padma-West); Lerab Drubpa (Karma-North); and Meri Barwa (Buddha-Center).

38. Guru Rinpoche, identical to our own teacher.

39. Tib. *rtsa;* Skt. *nāḍī*

40. Tib. *rlung;* Skt. *prāṇa*

41. Tib. *thig le;* Skt. *bindu*

42. The ground of all, or universal ground (Tib. *kun gzhi;* Skt. *ālaya*). Tulku Thondup writes, in *Enlightened Journey,* p. 204-207, "the karma of the universal ground is the karma that is stored in the universal ground or according to Khenpo Ngagchung, it is the karmas created by the consciousness of the universal ground, which has dualistic concepts (an intellectual obscuration) with traces."

43. Dilgo Khyentse Rinpoche says, above: "Through the blessing of the guru, our body, speech, and mind and the guru's enlightened body, speech, and mind will become indistinguishably one. Here, we simply remain in equipoise, within the state of emptiness and pure awareness." According to Jamyang Khyentse Chökyi Lodrö, if we cannot rest fully in that state at this point, we can recite the Vajra Guru mantra.

Selected Bibliography

Chagdud Tulku. *Gates to Buddhist Practice.* Junction City: Padma Publishing, 1993.

Chögyam Trungpa. *Heart of the Buddha.* Boston & London: Shambhala, 1991.

———. *The Lion's Roar.* Boston & London: Shambhala, 1992.

Dilgo Khyentse. *The Wish-Fulfilling Jewel: The Practice of Guru Yoga According to the Longchen Nyingthig Tradition.* Boston & London: Shambhala, 1988.

———. *The Excellent Path to Enlightenment.* Ithaca: Snow Lion, 1996.

———. *Enlightened Courage.* Ithaca: Snow Lion, 1993.

Dudjom Rinpoche. *The Nyingma School of Tibetan Buddhism.* Boston: Wisdom, 1992.

Jamgon Kongtrul. *The Torch of Certainty.* Boston and London: Shambhala, 1977.

Kalu Rinpoche. *The Dharma.* Albany: State University of New York Press, 1986.

Longchen Rabjam. *The Practice of Dzogchen.* Ithaca: Snow Lion, 1996.

———. *Dakini Teachings.* Boston & London: Shambhala, 1990.

Padmasambhava. *Advice from the Lotus-Born.* Boudhanath: Rangjung Yeshe Publications, 1994.

Patrul Rinpoche. *The Heart Treasure of the Enlightened Ones.* Boston & London: Shambhala, 1992.

———. *The Words of My Perfect Teacher.* San Francisco: HarperCollins, 1994.

Ricard, Matthieu. *Journey to Enlightenment.* New York: Aperture, 1996.

Sogyal Rinpoche. *Dzogchen and Padmasambhava.* Santa Cruz: Rigpa Publications, 1990.

———. *The Tibetan Book of Living and Dying.* San Francisco: Harper Collins, 1992.

Thinley Norbu. *The Small Golden Key.* Boston & London: Shambhala, 1993.

Tromge, Jane. *Ngöndro Commentary.* Junction City, Ca.: Padma Publishing, 1996.

Tulku Thondup. *The Dzogchen Preliminary Practice of the Innermost Essence.* Dharamsala: Library of Tibetan Works and Archives, 1982.

———. *Enlightened Journey.* Boston & London: Shambhala, 1995.

———. *Masters of Meditation and Miracles.* Boston & London: Shambhala, 1996.

Tulku Urgyen Rinpoche. *Repeating the Words of the Buddha.* Kathmandu: Rangjung Yeshe Publications, 1992.

Yeshe Tsogyal. *The Lotus Born.* Boston & London: Shambhala, 1993.

Index